Bad Habits Keeping You From Losing Weight

Key Habits to Help You Lose Weight Plus Tips on How to Stop Mindless Snacking and Eating With Your Emotions for Women

Yara Green

Dawn Publishing House

contained within this document, including, but not limited to, errors, omissions, or inaccuracies.

Table of Contents

Introduction

We all know that to lose weight we need to eat right and workout. Despite nearly everyone having this information more people are reported as overweight or obese each year. Why is it that we know what we should be doing, yet millions of us struggle to implement these two healthy-living factors?

If you are like millions of others, you do not have an answer. You know what you should do, yet you can't get yourself to do it or, at least, not consistently. So, like millions of others, you enlist in the help of a diet.

You choose one that promises fast weight loss. You cut back calories, forbid yourself from eating junk, and you even start working out. However, shortly after starting, you skip a workout here, let yourself have a little treat there, and soon you abandon your efforts.

Then, you start all over with a new diet promising fast results. The cycle has been going on for years.

You have probably been fighting with your weight for years. You are fed up with dieting. You lost the weight, or some of it, but gained it back, plus more. Starting another diet doesn't interest you because you refuse to deprive yourself of the foods you enjoy or waste hours at a gym feeling uncomfortable, insecure, and judged. There has to be a better, easier way.

Wouldn't it be nice to sit down at a meal and enjoy it from beginning to end? To savor the flavors and feel satisfied as you eat. To finish your meal without feeling weighed down, bloated, uncomfortable or sick? How much extra time and energy do you think you would gain if you didn't have to question what you were eating? How much more would you enjoy dining out, holiday parties, and home cooked meals if you got to eat what you wanted without feeling guilty?

The problem is, you have been approaching weight loss the wrong way. You are told to focus on what and how much you eat. You are told to workout for a certain amount of time so you burn calories and those burned calories would equal weight loss. Unfortunately, sticking to a limiting variety of food and working out when you are famished doesn't get you the lasting results you wish for.

Are you wondering if it is possible to just eat what you want without fretting over the carbs or fat you are consuming? Is it possible to look in the mirror and feel accepting of your reflection? You might have given up hope. You're just "big boned," or "everyone in your family is overweight, so you are too." You make excuses to ease the pain and try to accept that you are just destined to be overweight.

You do not have to make excuses any more. You do not have to go on another diet. And you do not have to workout excessively. What if you could get the weightloss results you have been dreaming of by making one small change to your day? What if you didn't have to give up your favorite foods or tell yourself you are not allowed that decadent dessert because you are trying to lose weight? You can!

I understand what you are going through. For years I was stuck yo-yo dieting, trying to lose weight fast, only to find myself a few months later back where I started. I would then force even further food restrictions on myself. I would tell myself I was going to go to the gym even more and workout for even longer. I was determined to lose weight. But my efforts were wasted. So I started researching the best weight loss plans around and found that every one of them was flawed. They all left out a key component to making a lifestyle change: mindset.

Most dieting books tell you what to eat, how much to eat, and forbidden foods. This book gives you examples of balanced meals and provides information on what your body needs, but there are no food restrictions in this book. That's right, if you want to eat your ice cream and cookies after dinner, go right ahead. This book will shine a new light on dieting and help you address the core problems with your eating habits that have been causing you to keep on that extra weight.

This book is designed to tackle the number one component that keeps people returning to old habits. Your mindset. The way you think about food, exercise, and other healthy habits needs to be reframed. You will learn how to reframe your thinking and rid yourself of the dieting mindset that often leads to more anxiety and weight gain rather than loss.

You will also learn that the best way to make a lifelong change is to start with one small thing. I mean, so small that you would ridicule yourself for failing not to do it, like having to do one sit-up or eating one piece of fruit a week. You will learn how this approach is one of the most effective ways to create lasting change and get your journey to a healthy lifestyle started.

Throughout this book, you will gain a deeper understanding of what drives your eating behaviors. You will find various tips, strategies, and exercises to combat some of the most common disordered eating patterns like mindless snacking, binge eating, and emotional eating. The focus is on addressing your eating behaviors so you can make permanent changes.

If you are looking for a quick fix to lose weight, you will not find it here. If you want to just drop a few pounds to fit into a dress for an upcoming event, or slim down to look good in a bikini, you aren't going to find that here. This book is not about reaching an ideal weight to look a certain way to feel good about yourself.

This book will provide a brand new perspective on how you view and treat your body. If you do not love yourself, it will be hard to stay committed to the changes you wish to make. Only through self-love will we begin to make choices that nurture our body. You will learn effective strategies to help you lose weight but the approach is different from what you read in other dieting books.

Be aware, not all the suggestions in this book are new or revolutionary. The difference between what you will learn here and what you have read elsewhere are the strategies to act upon the information you have. You will learn how to set effective goals, track your progress, and allow your body to guide you. If you are ready to break free of the endless dieting cycle and begin making changes that will last for the rest of your life, let's get started!

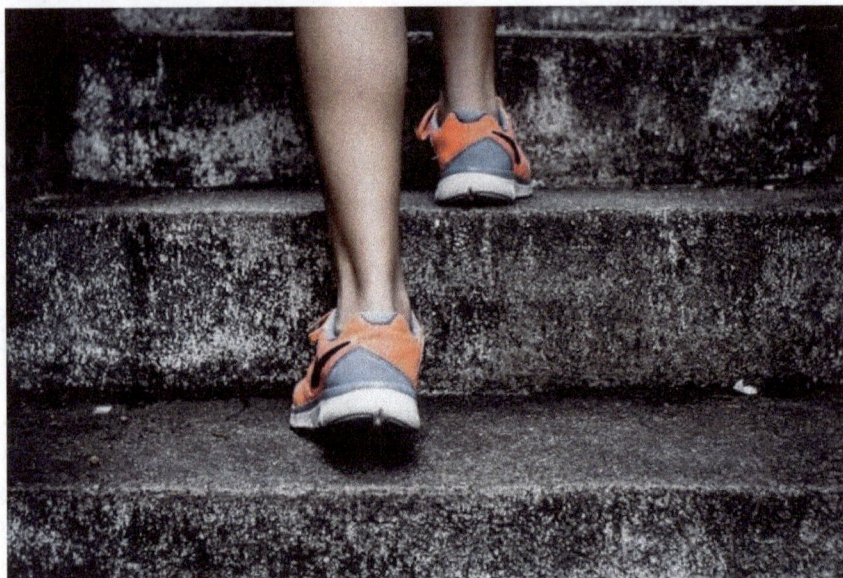

Chapter 1:

Never Diet Again

Weight loss diets are only a temporary fix for long-term problems. While they can be effective for losing weight, they are less effective for keeping weight off. How many diets have you been on? One, five, more—have you tried them all?

Maybe you haven't tried a traditional low-carb diet, but there is a good chance that you have a dieting mindset. How often do you second guess what you are going to eat because it has too much sugar or grease? How many times have you told yourself you need to lose weight to feel better about yourself? Nearly everyone lives with some aspects of a dieting mindset, and this is counterproductive to weight loss.

The diet industry thrives on people jumping from one diet to another. They promise fast weight loss but not permanent weight loss. This is why the diet industry is consistently one of the highest grossing industries year-after-year.

The promise of instant results without effort keeps millions jumping on board time and time again. The damage that constant dieting causes leaves many with disappointing results. It is important to understand why instant-result diets do not work as you begin to start adopting new habits that will result in long-lasting weight loss.

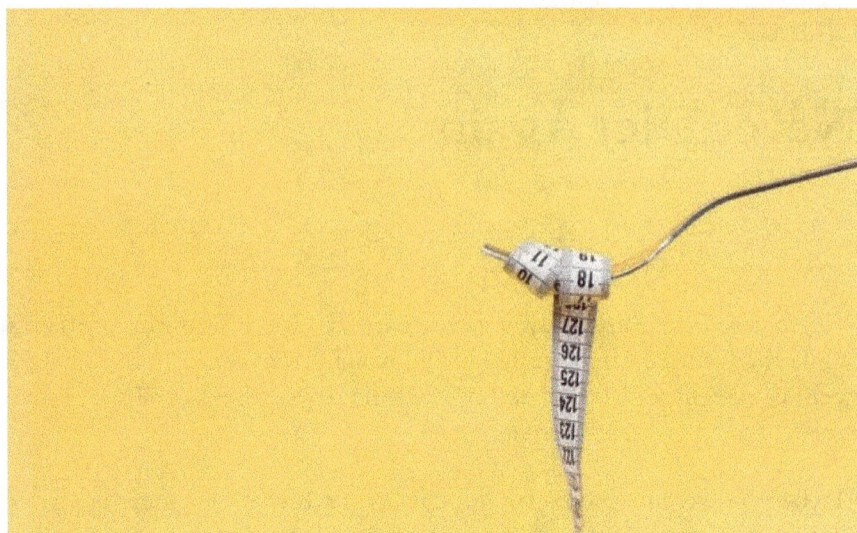

The Science Behind Dieting

The dieting industry is a billion-dollar industry that operates on body shaming and misconceptions. Consider all the shakes, bars, programs, supplements, and teas you see at the grocery store that promise rapid weight loss. How many commercials do you see for diet plans and programs that insist they are scientifically backed systems? Millions of people go from one diet scheme to the next without success and becoming more disappointed after each failed attempt.

Restrictive diets operate with outdated information that if we limit what and how much we eat, we will manage our weight with ease. If you are like me, you know there is nothing easy about sticking to a diet. But, we are bombarded with information that tells us we need to diet so we look a certain way or feel more energized. Everywhere you turn the diet culture is lurking making you feel guilty for eating a cupcake or clapping for you when you choose a salad.

Unfortunately, as creatures who crave instant gratification, we get sucked into new dieting promises time after time. We want to see results instantly without having to put much effort into losing the weight. When you take a close look at the dieting cycle, it is easy to see why you keep feeling like you fail each time.

Traditionally, diets encourage:

- Eating less than your body needs.

- Neglecting the body's natural hunger and fullness cues.

- Placing strict guidelines on what you can and cannot eat.

- Approaching physical activity as a means to burn calories and lose weight.

These actions are appealing because we feel we are controlling what influences our weight.

In reality, the feigned control causes more internal turmoil that leads to weight gain, rather than loss. We end up restricting what we eat to an unrealistic and unsustainable point . Eventually, whether it is a few days or a few weeks into the diet plan, we cave.

We let ourselves have one little cheat and we end up binging. After our out-of-control feeding frenzy we conclude that we need to be harder on ourselves. We need to place more limitations on what we eat and force ourselves to exercise even more. Then, the cycle repeats itself. Many who start on one diet find themselves stuck in this restriction-dysfunctional eating-restriction diet cycle for years. It is time to disrupt this cycle and begin focusing on what really initiates weight loss.

Why Diets Do Not Work

Restrictive diets focus on trying to control external factors, while completely neglecting our internal systems. There are a few key reasons why diets, although promoting weight loss, actually result in weight gain.

Diets Are Too Restrictive.

Nearly all diets have a list of foods to eat and foods not to eat. Some exclude whole food groups or forbid foods we love. While some dieters can stick to these restrictions for a few days, or even a few weeks, eventually we give into temptation. When we tell ourselves we are not allowed to have certain foods we begin to crave these foods more. The urges to consume become so intense that, when we do let ourselves indulge a little, we over consume and binge. After this overindulgence we either jump to the conclusion that the diet will not work or place even more restrictions on what we eat to avoid binging again. However, more restrictions only cause the binge cycle to start over.

You Are Forced to Make Too Many Changes All at Once.

When starting a diet we are expected to incorporate a number of new eating habits, new exercise, and follow specific 'rules' immediately, all at the same time. The problem is trying to change so many things all at once depletes our motivation. We may change a few things, but when we realize that we're not implementing everything, we become frustrated and discouraged. We slack off a little more until eventually we are back to eating how we have always eaten.

Diets Are Not Sustainable and We Lose Our Willpower to Stay Committed.

Our willpower is what controls our impulses. The more we stick to a diet the better we feel and the stronger our willpower remains. Over time, however, we begin to lose the motivation to maintain a diet plan. Our will power relies on our ability to make the best choices in the moment. The more choices we have to make, the more our will power depletes. When we lose the willpower to stick to the diet guidelines, we revert to old eating habits.

While diets give you a plan to follow they often cause you to second-guess your food choices. At the end of a stressful day are you really going to weigh the pros and cons of cutting up some vegetables and sitting down in front of a bowl of salad? Or are you going to reach in the fridge or stop at the fast food place to just feed yourself whatever is quick and easy?

Yo-Yo Dieting and Weight Gain

An average of 95% of people who go on a diet regain the weight loss, and often more, within one to five years (*Why diets do not work: How to avoid the dieting cycle and eat for your health*. 2019). This is true whether the person adheres to the diet within the five years or not. This statistic clearly indicates that diets do not work. However, that does not stop thousands of people from jumping on one diet after another.

Diets neglect and encourage us to ignore our body cues. We are instructed to eat a small amount which may leave us feeling hungry. Further restrictions may limit our intake of required nutrients. Putting our bodies through such chaos forces us into survival or famine mode.

Developed to stop starvation when we were hunter gatherers, in the famine mode, our body stores more fat when we do not regularly provide it with the fuel it needs. Jumping from one diet to the next puts excess stress on the body. Being stressed results in more cortisol being pumped into your body, which you will learn affects appetite in a negative way.

Uncertain when the next meal will be, our metabolism slows to preserve energy. A slower metabolism results in fewer calories burned throughout the day. When the body is in famine mode, it resorts to storing extra fat when it does receive food because it is uncertain when the next supply of energy will come and must store fat as an emergency energy source.

This famine mode underlies yo-yo dieting. You may lose weight initially, but it almost always is regained. You go on a diet again; because you got results the first round, you feel confident you will be able to lose the weight again.

The second round you do everything exactly the same, but it takes you twice along to lose the same amount of weight. But, here is the biggest shock factor: The time it takes for you to regain the weight occurs in half the time as before. For example, you stick to a diet and hit your goal weight in 30 days. It then took 60 days for you to notice you had regained the weight back. You go on a diet again, but it takes 60 days to lose the same amount of weight and just 30 days to gain it back this time.

The more yo-yo dieting you do, the more resistant your body is to losing weight. It will take more time and a lot more effort to keep losing the weight. In the long run, continuing with this cycle will result in regaining more weight than you initially had on your frame.

You Can't Just Focus on What You Eat

Diets only address what you eat, not why, how, where, or when you eat. While eating a well-balanced diet is essential to maintain a healthy body, there is much more to it than just putting food in your mouth and swallowing.

Eating is not just a physical act, there are emotions and hundreds of thoughts that come into play when we grab something to eat. Diets do not address the emotional or mental aspects of eating. These components of eating develop our eating habits and become deeply ingrained in our psyche.

Our relationship with food is centered around habits. We rarely allow our body to naturally guide us in deciding when, what, or why we eat. We seldom eat because we are actually hungry. This behavior has been taught to us from a young age.

As babies, we were in tune with our body. When we are hungry we cry and are fed. When we are full we simply refuse to eat more. As we grow, this behavior becomes unacceptable. We're told when to eat and warned, if we do not eat now, we will not eat again until the next meal. We're told what to eat and if we do not eat what is given, we're often punished by having been denied other food or special treats. Others portion how much we eat or we are often shamed for not cleaning our plate.

Other factors also distort our eating. News, media, and celebrities all flaunt attractive bodies that are thin and fit. We learn about their success with one diet and decide that is what we need to do to be flawless. They fail to mention the personal trainer or private chef that did most of the work for them: planning, shopping for, and preparing their meals; , crafting and guiding them through their exercise routine. Additionally, if these celebrities gain weight or stop restricting themselves and maintain their natural healthy weight, they are ridiculed.

There are plenty of problematic habits we have followed since childhood and never questioned or tried to change. We just automatically follow our habitual routine. But, habits can be modified, replaced, or stopped.

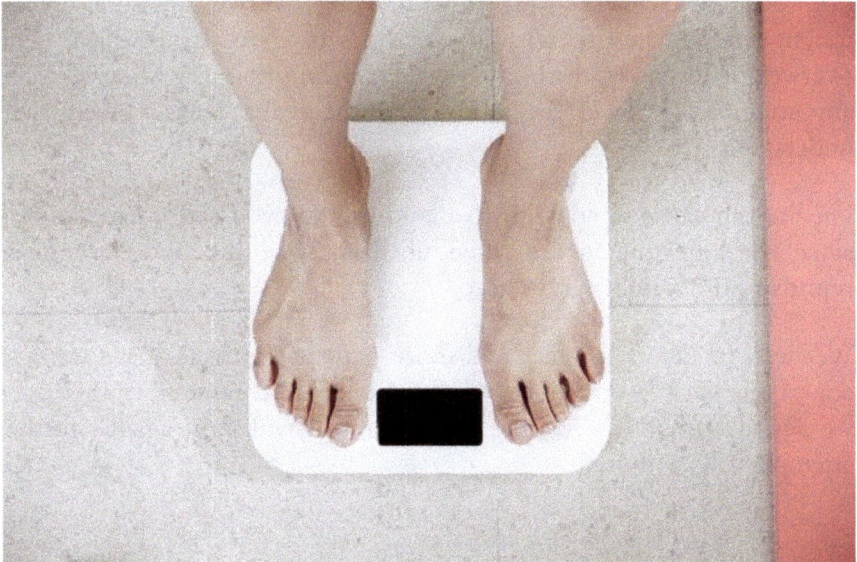

The Problem With The Scale

A misconception of diets is that to be healthy, we are supposed to be a particular weight. The main reason people begin to diet is because they, or someone else, feels they need to lose weight. While this may be true, the amount of required weight loss is often inaccurate.

Research is being conducted on 'healthy' weight and how much control we have over the scale. Many are preoccupied with dropping pounds and, when we do not see the weight coming off, we become frustrated and discouraged. New research indicates that your weight may have nothing to do with how healthy you are or if you are at greater risk for developing serious health complications because you are 'overweight'. If you eat a balanced, healthy diet, your body will naturally arrive at its ideal weight. It may fluctuate five or ten pounds but it has its own ideal weight. This weight may not be as low as you want it to be. It is the weight at which your body functions properly.

The number on the scale is not a reflection of how healthy you are. Get it out of your head that you need to be under a certain weight to be healthy and attractive.

For those who have struggled with being overweight, your natural weight has adjusted to what the body is used to. If you have been overweight for years, the body is used to being that weight; it will fight any attempts to lower the number on the scale. This is essential to understand.

Dieting can cause rapid adjustments to the way you eat or exercise but, since the adjustments are often unsustainable, the body eventually returns to the weight it is used to.

We need to take a steadier and more patient approach if we want to adjust our natural body weight. We also need to remember that once we get to our body's natural ideal weight, it will fight against further attempts to lose more.

Unfortunately, it is not enough to understand why diets do not work. Whether you have been on a diet or not, you likely have a dieting mindset that keeps you from achieving your weight loss goals. This is the main factor most people neglect when it comes to losing weight. You may be sabotaging your own efforts or letting external factors hold you back.

Chapter 2:

Adopting a New Mindset

To create healthy habits, you must change your behaviors. You will not change your behavior until you change your thoughts. To change our thoughts we need to believe that change is possible.

Adopting a new mindset is the secret weapon to losing weight and keeping it off. Many people neglect mindset when it comes to losing weight. They believe if they just follow a diet plan they will lose weight. However, they fail to address the issues with their current eating patterns and once reaching their goal weight, they return to the unaddressed, flawed eating patterns.

Many factors contribute to having an unhealthy relationship with eating and food. They are all rooted in our thoughts and learnings about food.

We need to reword what we say and believe so we are motivated to stick to new eating habits. You must change your mindset. Without the right mindset, you will give into temptation and return to old habits that cause you to suffer and struggle with your weight.

Good and Bad Foods

You do not have to choose between that decadent chocolate cake or steamed broccoli, you can have both. A key to embracing a new way of eating is to allow yourself to eat and enjoy your food. Categorizing food as good or bad promotes shame and guilt about how we feel after we eat. Instead, we must see all food as good and, instead, tune into how we physically feel when we eat rather than our emotions.

Denying yourself of foods you enjoy will only increase the risk of binging or overeating. When we overindulge we often berate ourselves for lack of control. The overindulgence has nothing to do with control.

The more restrictions we place on ourselves the more we will think about and crave those things. This is true for anything. Consider a time when you told yourself you were no longer going to do something. Maybe you only had two drinks when you were out with your friends. Or you told yourself you would buy only one pair of shoes or one new shirt. When you limit yourself, how often do you think about the thing you said you wouldn't buy or enjoy? How many times do you notice images or conversation about these things? When we place restrictions on ourselves and try to ignore them we actually draw more attention to them. The same goes with food, but to a greater extent.

Consider the last time you successfully followed a diet program for a few weeks. You were probably proud of your progress and discipline. You were losing weight and you didn't feel ashamed of eating your meals in front of anyone because they consisted of 'good' foods.

Then, you attended a party, had a night out with friends, or maybe the holidays started. There were treats, chips, salsa, ice cream, and other 'bad' foods you aren't allowed to eat. How much of your time was spent convincing yourself to stay on your diet programs? You probably had a hard time enjoying the event because you spent so much time fighting to avoid the temptations. If you did give in, you went all in. You told yourself that you had either been doing so well on your diet that you deserve a reward or you had already blown your diet so you might as well enjoy all you can. Neither of these mindsets promote a healthier way of eating.

The more we tell ourselves to avoid eating something because it is bad, the more we crave it. After we give in, we feel like we have failed ourselves. But, it is not just the temptation that makes it hard to resist, our bodies are out of sync.

Restricting your food intake or cutting out food groups can alter the hunger and fullness hormones. You may become hungrier because your body is not getting what it needs. In addition, the fullness hormones that tell you to stop eating are released more slowly. This leads you to overeat more often. It is why you can eat everything in sight and still feel hungry despite having no more room in your stomach to put anything else.

Dieting also slows down your metabolism. This is especially true when you restrict calorie intake or cut out essential food groups. The body goes into famine, or starvation, mode when required nutrients are restricted. In famine mode, the body will do what it must to conserve energy. Your metabolism slows down if you do not use up more energy than necessary throughout the day. A healthy metabolism is essential for weight loss. When it slows down, you will burn fewer calories and may gain weight rather than lose it.

Yo-yo dieting shifts your body's natural hunger rhythms. Instead of craving and adding fuel every few hours, diet schedules train you to load up on a lot of fuel all at once and store a majority of it for later use. This is why you find yourself overeating when you do eat. The body is preparing for another famine so it triggers you to keep eating to ensure it has enough fuel to use now and plenty in storage for later.

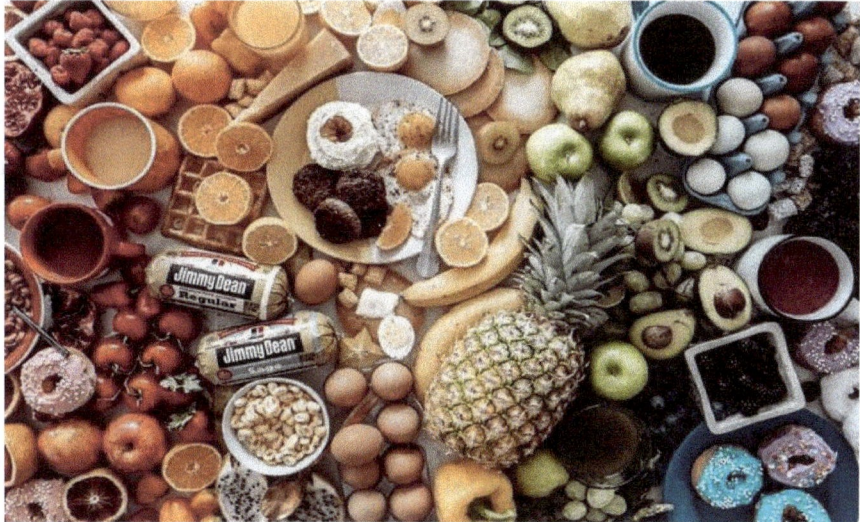

Rid Yourself of the Dieting Mindset

The dieting mindset connects your self-worth with your food choices. If you eat foods that are 'bad,' you feel bad, weak, or unworthy of being healthy. This thinking encourages emotional and binge eating. Instead of falling prey to this type of thinking, shift your focus.

Recognizing when the dieting mindset is at play is difficult at times. Many external factors support a dieting mindset. For so long, we hear the same phrase about food that we just naturally take them on as truth. Some of dieting mindset thoughts appear harmless:

- "I shouldn't eat that doughnut because it is bad for me."

- "That milkshake has too much sugar."

- "I already ate enough carbs today".

These phrases seem to reinforce better food choices but they are shame-loaded messages that make you feel bad for wanting to enjoy your desserts and treats. But, you can enjoy all foods, without shame and guilt.

Instead of categorizing foods as good or bad and micromanaging them, shift your thoughts slightly. Instead of saying "That big slice of cake is going to make you fat," or "That big slice of cake has too much sugar," we can tell ourselves, "If I have one small slice of cake I will enjoy it more than if I had a large piece. That larger piece of cake is going to make me feel lethargic and uncomfortable."

This subtle shift in your thinking about the cake does not forbid you from having it. Instead, you are making yourself aware of how that cake is going to make you feel after you eat it. You are allowing yourself to eat the cake, but you are encouraging self-control to eat only what you know you are going to enjoy. This takes practice to implement every time and there may be times when you decide, "I know I am going to regret eating this because I am going to feel sick, but I am eating it anyways." If this happens, do not beat yourself up and continue to binge, realize that your thought indicates a greater sense of awareness, which *is* progress. The more you shift your thoughts about your food intake, and allow yourself to eat any foods, the easier it will become to eat what you enjoy in moderation. Over time, you may find that the urge to eat the cake starts to disappear.

Think of 'More'

Reframe your thoughts to focus on the 'more' you should have. When constantly reminding yourself of the foods to remove from your diet, you feel deprived. You have to eat fewer calories to lose weight (or use more than you eat). Thus, you must cut back on something we eat. A restrictive approach to eating immediately increases cravings. Thus, you can't focus on what you are cutting back on or limiting in your diet.

Instead, focus on the foods you are eating more. You get to eat as many vegetables as you want, without limitation. You can enjoy more sweet and tasty fruit. When you shift our focus from what you can have less of to what you can have more of, you minimize feelings of deprecation.

Also combine this 'more' mindset to how you feel. You will feel more energized due to eating all those fruits and vegetables. You are going to be more confident, more healthy, more motivated. You will not be bothered by those other things you are eating as much when you are more focused on what you are gaining rather than missing.

Negative Self-Talk

While dieting causes turmoil with our body's natural system, it is ultimately the way we talk to ourselves which can dictate our weight loss outcomes. If we riddle ourselves with negativity, shame, and disgust around how we look, we aren't going to experience the transformation we desire. If we constantly feel guilty for eating certain foods or not sticking with a diet, we are setting ourselves up for failure.

Be aware of how the dieting culture has overwhelmed your thought processes, which does not only include thoughts about food. Thinking you need to look a certain way, hating your pant size, or feeling shame about anything else about your body are all driven by the diet culture, and all support negative self-talk.

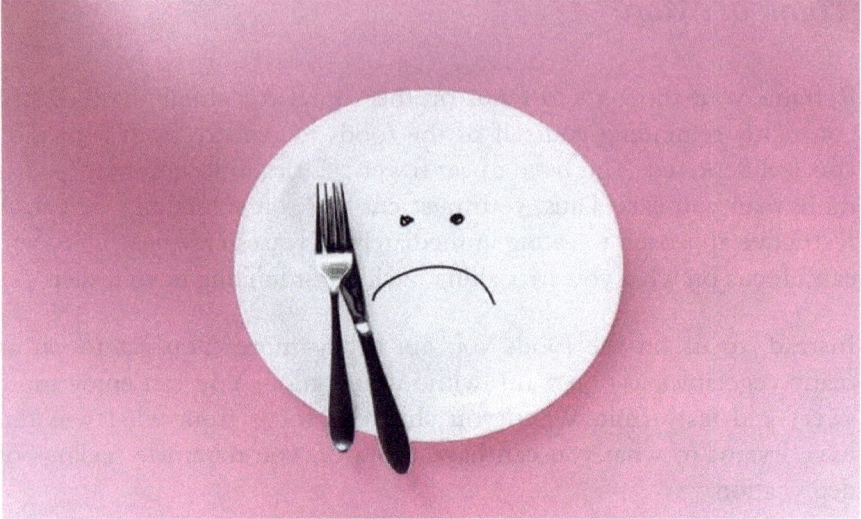

Reframing What You Think and Say

A big mindset struggle that many face when changing habits is changing what we already do automatically. Creating new habits takes a lot of effort but eventually the change will become automatic. Unfortunately, our brains are hardwired to repeat things we have done before and that are easy because they require less energy.

To accommodate our brains' needs to stay comfortable, we need to adopt a more positive outlook about the things we commit to doing. For example, exercise is one of the hardest habits for many to adopt. Working out is good for us but it is hard and takes a lot of effort. As soon as we think, *I need to workout*, the thought is often immediately followed by another, *I hate working out*.

A negative attitude toward exercise makes it hard to get motivated and moving. Again, if you make a subtle shift in your thinking, you can minimize the resistance to exercise. Try telling yourself *I get to move my body* or *I love that my body is strong because I workout*. We dive deeper into how to create exercising habits later on in the book, but keep this example in mind when you notice your thoughts resisting the changes you want to make.

To reframe thinking, you need to focus on the healthy habits you are adopting. Are you drinking more water? Are you sticking to an eating schedule instead of grazing all day? Have you started taking a short walk in the evening to unwind? When you begin to hear the negative chatter in your head, remind yourself of the changes you are making that will have a positive impact for the long-term. Remind yourself of these positive changes every day.

Focus on both the foods you can eat more of and the beneficial habits you are adopting. Even if it is one small change at a time, these changes will add up to big results. We all need to start somewhere, whether that is drinking an extra glass of water every day or going for a five-minute walk in the evening. Do not discredit your efforts or think that the small changes are not important. Recognize that small changes in behavior are habits changes, each one will ensure a healthier and happier future.

Creating a New Vision for Yourself

The body will change when your thoughts change, but it will not happen overnight. Many people become impatient when they are trying to lose weight or reach better health. What you need to remember is that you did not gain the extra weight overnight. If you eat a gourmet, five-course dinner the night before, you do not wake up spontaneously weighing fifteen pounds more than you did the day before. Do not expect to shed excess weight overnight or by making an occasional adjustment to a single habit. Improving your health is a process and enjoying the process helps you be successful and appreciate it even more in the future.

Hating yourself or your body doesn't lead to lasting change. You need to heal your relationship with yourself, your food, and your activities. Only when we can show ourselves love will we find a new reason to make the necessary changes to live a healthier lifestyle. Through love, we commit to nourishing our body and doing more of the things that keep it working in optimal health.

It is time to create a new vision of yourself. One that showcases all the amazing things your body has done for you, and will continue to do for you, if you learn to respect, nourish, and love it. Your body is designed specifically to function the way it needs to.

Each new habit you adopt will become a part of your new identity. As you begin to create these habits, remind yourself that you are simply the type of person that does them. For example you can say:

- *I am the type of person that drinks 90 ounces of water everyday.*

- *I am the type of person who workouts regularly.*

- *I am the type of person that prioritizes sleep.*

When you frame your thoughts in this way, your brain will naturally look for evidence in your day to support them. It does not matter if these phrases are 100% true or not in the present moment. Our brains can not distinguish between certain thoughts as being reality or as mini-motivations to encourage change. The brain will simply begin to look for evidence to support the thought.

Each time you are met with a decision about what to eat, whether to exercise, or loving and caring for yourself, ask yourself if you are the type of person that does one thing or the other. For example, *Am I a person who eats a sweet pastry for breakfast or am I a person that starts their day with a well-balanced breakfast of oats and fruits?* You get to decide what you want but your choice should reflect the new vision you have of yourself.

Chapter 3:

Getting In-Tune With Your Body

Once you begin to work on your mindset, you need to continue to heal your relationship with your body. You need to trust that it is telling you what it needs, when it needs it. Many eating habits can keep you out of touch with what your body needs. This is the main reason for overeating and getting sucked into binge eating cycles. For years, you have been ignoring what your body needs and have even been punishing yourself for listening to it.

It is time to tune into your body and relearn how to recognize its cues. When you honor your body's signs, you minimize your urges to binge or overeat. Honoring these cues heals your relationship with your body and it begins to trust you. Remember, if you have been dieting your body has gotten used to being in starvation mode, we need to reprogram it to be in fulfilled or satiated mode.

Although your body naturally signals what it needs, keep in mind that recognizing and acting on those cues can be a challenging process. Some people have difficulty recognizing hunger cues because they have ignored them for so long. At times, learning to understand the cues of your body can feel uncomfortable. You may hesitate to eat when you start to feel hungry because you believe you should still be full from your last meal. Keep in mind, if you have been dieting frequently, your body will need time to adjust and to trust that it will be nourished when it sends signals for food. Be patient, and trust your body.

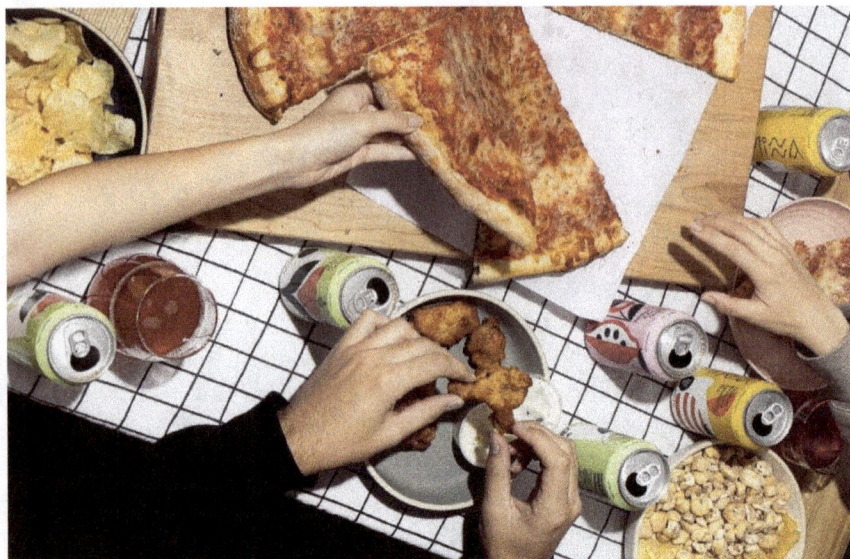

Understanding Your Eating Habits

Our eating habits begin to take shape in early childhood and will influence how we eat throughout our lives. There are many situations that can cause dysfunctional eating patterns,of which many you may be unaware. You can begin to identify the root causes of why you eat too much, not enough, or unbalanced meals by understanding your own eating habits.

First, you need to clarify your current habits. Take some time now to write out answers the following questions:

- How many meals do you have each day?
- How often do you snack throughout the day?
- What foods do you typically eat?
- Where do you eat?
- Do you typically eat on the go?

- How much do you eat? Do you often continue to eat even though you are full?

- What do you drink throughout the day?

- Is there anything about eating that causes you to feel anxious?

- Do you have to clear your plate?

- Do you force yourself to eat certain foods?

- Do you have to fill your plate or do you restrict yourself to a small portion of food?

- Do you regularly skip meals?

- How often do you find yourself eating late at night?

- How often do you wait until you feel as though you are starving to eat?

- Do you eat around others? If so, who? If not, why?

- When do you find yourself eating when you are not hungry?

As you write, your answers will provide insight into how factors from your past contribute to disordered eating patterns that you can change. It is important that you are honest in your answers and that you take the time to consider the answer you write.

Childhood Habits

Parents unintentionally encourage poor eating habits in children and it is likely that you are struggling with your weight because of the habits they demonstrated for you. Even if your parents did not instill the following ideas on you, you may have been exposed to these habits from others.

Your Parents Controlled When and What You Ate.

Most families stick to eating schedules that consider the adults' needs but rarely the children's. If a parent works early in the evening, dinner is moved up. It doesn't matter if the children are hungry at this time or not, they are expected to sit down and eat. Additionally, not many families let their kids help with planning meals. They are told what to eat and they must eat it, even if they do not like it.

Parents who tell their kids when and what to eat are teaching their kids to ignore their natural hunger and satiation cues. During infancy these two signals are strong and parents react to them appropriately. When the baby screams, they are fed, when they have had enough the baby refuses to eat. Parents do not argue with these behaviors, but as a child grows older, parents take control.

These children become adults who do not recognize when they are hungry or full. They will often wait until they have reached starvation to eat and then go through a binging episode in which they overeat. They will often avoid certain foods as well, either because they were forced to eat them when they were younger and have a negative attitude about the foods or because they were told they were bad foods and not to eat them.

If you notice that you are rigid with when, what, and how much you eat, you may be suffering from these childhood habits. It is essential that you begin to listen to your natural cues. Learn to enjoy your food fully, including how it tastes and how it makes you feel. Finally, it is important that you begin to feed your body when you get the first cues of hunger, even if it is a small snack to hold you over until your next meal. We cover each of these body cue factors more thoroughly throughout this chapter.

There Was Emphasis on Weight Gain Due to What You Ate.

Some parents try to control their child's weight if there is the slightest gain. Some parents weigh their children and even put them on restrictive diets starting at a young age. As we have covered, food restriction causes dysfunctional eating that will carry over into adulthood. In addition, placing so much emphasis on body image at such a young age develops children who have a negative view of the way they look.

If you notice that you are constantly worried about gaining weight and put extreme restrictions on what and how much you eat, this is commonly due to having a poor body image. Understand that your weight naturally fluctuates. While gaining an excessive amount of weight should be a concern, a few pounds is nothing to worry about. To correct poor eating habits associated with the fear of gaining weight, you need to mend the relationship you have with your body. You need to recognize the unrealistic views of maintaining the perfect weight or fitting into a specific size. Learn to appreciate your body, even when it is a little heavier.

You Heard the Word 'Fat' Frequently.

The word 'fat' is weighed down with many negative views. You may have heard your parents or others use 'fat' to describe someone they were fond of but who they thought was lazy or lacked direction in life. You may have developed a distorted view of yourself and may be overly concerned with how you look. On top of this, you may have an underlying fear or worry about being judged by others—or you may be quick to judge others—by their body or weight. This mindset fuels a need to constantly be on a diet.

When the word fat is constantly used in connection with negative traits, like being lazy or disorganized, we associate the negativity with the body image and can begin to adopt a negative view of ourselves. For example, if you are not meeting the real or perceived expectation of others, you may consider yourself fat and lazy. If your home is not neat and tidy, you may believe your are a fat slob. This is a distorted view influenced by how the word was used as you grew up.

If you find yourself referring to yourself or others as fat you need to look at the facts of the situation. Someone's size, just as your size, should not be a measurement of what type of person they are. Make an effort to notice other qualities or characteristics that have nothing to do with weight.

Food was Hidden, Forbidden, or Taken Away.

If your parents constantly worried about you overeating, you may have grown guilt about how much you eat. Some parents will hide food to ensure that their children aren't eating outside of planned meals. This results in children developing a food scarcity mindset. You might have forced yourself to eat even when you were not hungry for fear of the food being taken away and not getting a chance to eat again. Likewise, if certain foods were forbidden because they were not good for you, you may overindulge in them as an adult.

You might not regularly notice how this impacts your eating patterns but you may find that you have a need to constantly have an overabundance of food in your home. So much that a lot of it might go to waste.

You might also still experience this scarcity fear especially when dining with your parents. Do you notice at family meals that you become more anxious about how much you eat?

Address this mindset by reframing your fears. Once you can reassure yourself that you do not have to worry about when and where your next meal is, you can permit yourself to eat when you are hungry without fear of never eating again. Many adults with this fear will ignore their hunger cues and wait to eat, which often leads to overeating or binging later.

You Were Told Certain Foods Were Good and Others Were Bad.

Although well-meaning, parents who teach their kids that certain foods are bad and others good cause children to develop judgments about what they eat. As discussed, this often translates to a negative identity when you do eat this bad food. If you were constantly told not to eat sugary foods, fried foods, or snacks because they are bad, you probably have a conflict in which you wait to enjoy those foods but then feel shame for doing so.

Instead of labeling foods as 'bad,' using a new label such as 'sometimes' or 'fun' foods begins to eliminate the negative feelings you have when eating them. Remind yourself that certain foods like lean protein, fruits, and vegetables are essential for staying healthy; other foods may not be as beneficial, but can still be eaten.

One or Both of Your Parents Were Always on a Diet.

Many children grow up hearing about one or both parents being on a diet or needing to lose weight. You may have watched your mom look at herself disappointingly as she pinched at her waist or talked about needing to lose a few pounds to fit into a certain dress or pants. Children who are exposed to this behavior regularly tend to view this as normal. They grow up thinking that dieting is necessary and this belief can cause a variety of disordered eating patterns.

If you were constantly exposed to the dieting mindset as a child, it is more likely that you obsess over what and how much you eat. You may also take additional extreme measures like overexercising to combat weight gain. You need to develop a new approach to eating that focuses on eating well-balanced meals. Also, remember that your body is designed to be a certain way. Not everyone is meant to be tall and stick thin. Do not compare the way you look to others, learn to love your body and accept it for the way it is because that is what it was designed to serve you.

You Were Punished for Not Eating Everything on Your Plate.

This is one of the most common, and inappropriate, eating habits children experience. I know plenty of adults who grew up in a home that was part of the "clean your plate club."

If you do not eat everything on your plate, you are forced to sit at the table until you do or until it is time for bed. If you do not finish everything on your plate, you are deprived of dessert or participating in evening activities. Some parents use guilt tactics to get their children to eat everything on their plate by mentioning there are other children starving around the world who would be grateful to have a meal like the one being wasted.

If you constantly feel you need to finish everything on your plate, no matter how full you are, this may be from having to clean your plate as a child. It is common for children who grew up in a home like this to be overweight and struggle more with weight management. To combat this flawed eating pattern, learn to recognize when you are full and allow yourself to stop eating. You can always save what you haven't eaten for later.

What Your Body Really Needs

The distorted eating patterns in the previous section have taught you to focus on the wrong things when eating. To change these eating habits you need to understand what your body needs and learn to listen to its cues. If you grew up in a home that encouraged inappropriate eating patterns, you have tuned out your body's natural signals.. Learning to recognize and respond to these cues again (like you did as a baby) is essential for weight loss.

The body needs the right balance of nutrients. Many diets that tell you to stop eating certain food groups often ignore the fact that the body relies on all five food groups for energy, vitamins, and minerals. When you learn what your body needs you can make better decisions about what and how much you eat. When you begin to nourish your body properly, your cravings for certain foods and urges to overeat will diminish.

This section is not telling you what you should or should not eat. The information here does not form rules or restrictions to follow when you eat. Refer to this section to balance your meals in an extra effort to keep your body healthy. Remember, you do not have to choose to eat just these foods and give up other things like cookies, chips, and candy. When you stop forbidding yourself from certain foods, your desire to consume them diminishes. Until this occurs, create a way that you can have both without guilt or self-punishment!

Macronutrients

Macronutrients need to be consumed in higher quantities. They are essential for supplying the body with sufficient energy, maintaining metabolism, and keeping the body functioning optimally.

Carbohydrates

Carbohydrates (carbs) are often misunderstood. Many people blame carbohydrate for excessive weight gain. This is because carbohydrates contain a significant amount of calories. While some forms of carbs are proven to add to weight, others are an essential source of fuel for the body.

Carbohydrates consist of:

- vegetables (starchy vegetables like potatoes and corn contain more carbs then non-starchy vegetables)
- rice
- sugar
- bread
- pasta
- beans
- fruits

The body gets nearly 65% of its energy from carbohydrates (The Open University n.d.). When we consume carbohydrates, the digestive system breaks them down into glucose, which is then absorbed into the bloodstream to provide energy to all our cells, tissues, and muscles. If we take in more carbohydrates than the body needs, the excess is stored away as fat so that it can be tapped into later.

It is important to know that there are three different groups of carbohydrates:

- monosaccharides
- disaccharides
- polysaccharides

Monosaccharides and disaccharides are considered simple carbs. When we consume these carbs, little digestion is necessary before they can be absorbed by the blood stream and the body quickly processes them and uses them for fuel. If we consume these in excess, there is a drastic spike in blood sugar levels and the body gets overwhelmed with sugar. All types of sugar, honey, and many sweet fruits consist of monosaccharides and disaccharides.

Polysaccharides are complex carbs. When we consume these carbs, the sugars cannot immediately be absorbed in the bloodstream and must be broken t down into simple sugars before they can be distributed throughout the body. This is a longer process and results in a steady stream of energy being released over a longer period of time. Starchy vegetables and whole grains are two examples of complex carbs.

There is also fiber, which is considered a carbohydrate. Unlike other forms of carbs, the body cannot break down fiber into simple sugars to use as fuel. Fiber remains undigested by the body. However, fiber affects the way the body releases and absorbs other carbohydrates. Fiber takes longer to pass through the digestive system than other carbs, which slows down the digestion of the other foods you consume with or after it. This slower digestion results in the sugar molecules being released slowly and reduces blood sugar spikes.

This is important to understand. For example, whole fruits consist of fast acting carbohydrates, but most also contain a significant amount of fiber. Fruit juices, on the other hand, have simple carbohydrates but the juicing of the fruit has removed the fiber. When you eat an apple, the fiber content slows down the release of the sugars in the apple. Blood sugar will often not spike as rapidly as if you drink the fruit juice. Eating an apple provides a steady stream of fuel instead of one quick jolt of energy the juice provides.

Unfortunately, traditional western diets consist primarily of simple carbohydrates that get quickly released and absorbed by the body. Processed sugar and flour are two of the most common culprits. Most people consume these frequently and it results in a consistent stream of excess energy that ends up being stored right away as fat. We often fail to allow enough time between carbohydrate intakes to tap our reserves so the fat doesn't get burned and we gain more and more weight.

Protein

Our body needs a supply of efficient protein to help promote cell growth and to build lean muscle. The immune system also relies on protein to function properly. It can also supply the body with energy when we do not consume enough carbohydrates. Between 10 and 35% of our calorie intake needs to come from viable protein sources (The Open University, n.d.). Quality proteins include lean meats, poultry, fish, eggs, milk, and cheese. There are also plant-based proteins such as beans, nuts, and legumes that contain less protein than animal sources, but plant-based sources often contain minerals and vitamins than animal proteins.

We need to consume high-quality proteins. Many overconsume poor-quality sources such as hot dogs, sausage, low-grade ground beef, and other processed meats that supply little protein and high amounts of saturated fats.

Fats

Like carbohydrates, fats also have a bad reputation. Fats can help or hinder body functionality. Fats provide the body with fatty acids and are essential for the absorption of vitamins A,D, E, and other fat-soluble vitamins.

There are two many types of fats:

- saturated

- unsaturated

Saturated fats are tightly packed fats that are not easily broken down by the intestines during digestion. When distributed throughout the body saturated fat builds up as plaque in the arteries. These fats cause higher levels of low density lipoproteins (LDL) in the bloodstream. High LDL cholesterol levels increase the risk of heart disease. Fatty meats like pork, processed meats, and refined oils contain high quantities of saturated fats.

Unsaturated fats are loosely packed fats, which allow enzymes to begin breaking them down as soon as they enter our mouth. When these fats reach the digestive track the amino acids are released through the body to help maintain cellular and muscular growth. There are two main types of unsaturated fats: monounsaturated and polyunsaturated.

 Monounsaturated fats are commonly derived from plant-based sources and are usually consumed as an oil, like olive or avocado oil. Polyunsaturated fats are omega-3 and omega-6 fatty acids. Omega-3 fatty acids are essential for heart and brain health. The best sources of omega-3s come from fish, flax seed, and chia seeds. Omega-6 fatty acids are essential for overall health but when consumed in high quantities can increase inflammation in the body and increase the risk of obesity. The most common sources of omega-6 are soybeans, canola, and sunflower oil.

We should be consuming more omega-3 fatty acids than omega-6 fatty acids. Fat should only make up around 20% of our daily calorie intake and a majority of this should come from unsaturated fat as opposed to saturated fats (The Open University, n.d.). However, most people do not eat the appropriate amount or type of fats. Most eat an excessive amount of fat, in general, and consume primarily saturated rather than unsaturated fats.

Everything we consume has a mixture of nutrients. Most foods are a great source of one or two macronutrients and will provide a handful of micronutrients. Foods are often categorized by the nutrient they are the most abundant in. For example, most fruits are considered carbohydrates because they have high sugar and fiber levels, but they also contain a wide variety of vitamins and minerals.

There are some exceptions to categorizing by the highest level of macronutrients. Black beans, for example, are often classed as plant protein but they contain more carbohydrates than protein. Although technically a carbohydrate, many people use them in place of animal proteins as their main source of protein (particularly vegans and vegetarians).

Micronutrients

Micronutrients include vitamins and minerals that we need to function. Some are essential because the body does not produce them naturally and we must get them through our diet; some essential vitamins and minerals are important because they are needed to help the body absorb specific vitamins and minerals. For example, our bodies do not produce magnesium on its own but we need this mineral to better absorb vitamin D better. Thus, we need to consume magnesium to properly utilize Vitamin D.

Vitamins are categorized as water-soluble or fat-soluble. Water-soluble vitamins are released directly into the bloodstream from the foods we consume. These vitamins easily move about the body and excesses of water-soluble vitamins are removed from the body by our kidneys. Water-soluble vitamins the body cannot be stored in our bodies to use later so we must have a consistent supply of them. Water-soluble vitamins perform many functions but, most importantly, they aid in digesting food, releasing food energy, and producing energy so the body functions properly.

Fat-soluble vitamins need to be transported throughout the body via carrier proteins. These types of vitamins can only access the bloodstream through lymph channels in the intestinal walls. The liver and fat tissues help store excess fat-soluble vitamins that can be released when needed. Since these vitamins can be stored you do not need to consume them daily, often you can consume them once a week and still have sufficient to supply the body with what it needs.

There are 13 essential vitamins the body needs (nine are part of the B vitamin family):

- Vitamin A (fat-soluble)

- Vitamin C (water-soluble)

- Vitamin D (fat-soluble)

- Vitamin E (fat-soluble)

- Vitamin K (fat-soluble)

- B Vitamins (water-soluble):

    o B1 Thiamin

    o B2 Riboflavin

    o B3 Niacin

    o B5 Pantothenic acid

    o B6

    o B7 Biotin

    o B9 Folic acid

    o Folate

    o B12

Most of these vitamins need to be replenished every two to three days. Some, like vitamin B12, can be stored in the body for several days or even years. We can supply the body with a majority of these vitamins by eating various fruits and vegetables.

Aside from the essential vitamins there are major and trace minerals the body needs. Some minerals can travel freely throughout the body and others rely on a carrier for transport or to help the necessary cells to absorb it.

Major minerals are essential to maintain proper water levels in the body, keep bones strong and healthy, and assist in stabilizing protein structures, like those that make up our hair and skin. Trace minerals are responsible for various tasks throughout the body. Some help transport oxygen, others boost the immune system, and some assist major minerals in strengthening bones. We need to maintain the proper balance of major and trace minerals. Having too much of one can create a deficiency in another. For example, if you have too much manganese this can cause an iron deficiency.

Additionally, we cannot produce certain hormones when we lack certain minerals. For example, consuming too little iodine hinders the production of thyroid hormones, which can lead to weight gain and a slower metabolism.

There are 16 essential minerals the body needs include:

- calcium (major)
- chloride (major)
- chromium (trace)
- copper (trace)
- fluoride (trace)
- iodine (trace)
- iron (trace)
- magnesium (major)
- manganese (trace)
- molybdenum (trace)
- phosphorus (major)
- potassium (major)
- selenium (trace)

- sodium (major)

- sulfur (major)

- zinc (trace)

We can get sufficient minerals from the foods we eat without having to worry about taking a supplement. However, we need to eat a balanced diet that includes fruits, vegetables, and lean proteins to ensure we are getting all the minerals our body needs.

Water

Water is vital for proper health and survival. Our body consists of water and nearly every organ, cell, tissues, and process the body performs is either made up of water or relies on water to operate. Whereas the body can survive for a few weeks without food, it can only last a few days without water.

There are conflicting recommendations about how much water one needs to drink. The traditional recommendation is to drink eight, eight-ounce glasses of water daily, which totals 64 ounces. Others suggest drinking half your body weight in ounces of water. For example, if you weigh 180 pounds then your goal should be to drink 90 ounces of water a day. There are others who suggest you need two to three liters or 67 to 100 ounces of water a day (The Open University, n.d.).

We can get some of our water intake from foods we eat. Watermelon, celery, and cucumbers all contain high quantities of water but are not normally heavily consumed. We cannot get the essential amount of water from food alone. But, most people are barely drinking half or even a quarter of any of the above recommendations. While most beverages like juice and tea do contain water, the amount is not substantial enough to fulfill our water requirements. Water must be consumed daily to maintain health.

Body Processes and Natural Rhythms

The body operates by following a variety of internal systems or circadian rhythms, meaning certain processes repeat a similar pattern every 24 hours. The most well-known circadian rhythm is our sleep-wake cycle, but there are also cycles associated with our brain function, metabolism, and appetite.

Light plays an integral part in regulating our circadian rhythm. What we eat, when we eat, and how much we eat can impair our internal clocks and cause them to become out of sync with one another. When we diet we run the risk of disrupting our body's internal clock because we are ignoring its natural rhythm .

When we eat, signals are sent to various organs that it is time to get active. The heart, liver, kidneys, and muscles all play a part in proper digestion. Eating switches the body into active mode because we use up a lot of energy through the digestive process. If you struggle to fall asleep in the evening, consider when your last meal was. Many people struggle to get to sleep when they eat too close to their bedtime because the body is still active. Darkness triggers the body to go into rest mode but because it is still digesting it can't. This begins to disrupt the activation of other systems and will cause some to become active before they should be.

It is possible to correct our systems and get our clocks aligned. Sticking to a mealtime schedule is one of the best ways to begin syncing your clocks so they work with each other. Going to bed and waking up at the same time every day is essential to keep our rhythms on track. Aim to eat your last meal at least two hours before your bedtime. This gives your body time to transition to its resting phase instead of digestion phase.

Even if your work schedule does not allow you to stick to a consistent routines or cyclers, there are still ways you can keep your clocks in check. For starters, keep your meal consumption to the daytime or light hours. Instead of trying to squeeze in three big meals, plan for several small meals while it is still light out. Ensure these meals are packed with fiber and include lean protein to help combat cravings. If you become tired, the body will want sugar and fat, eating fiber and protein will stop those cravings.

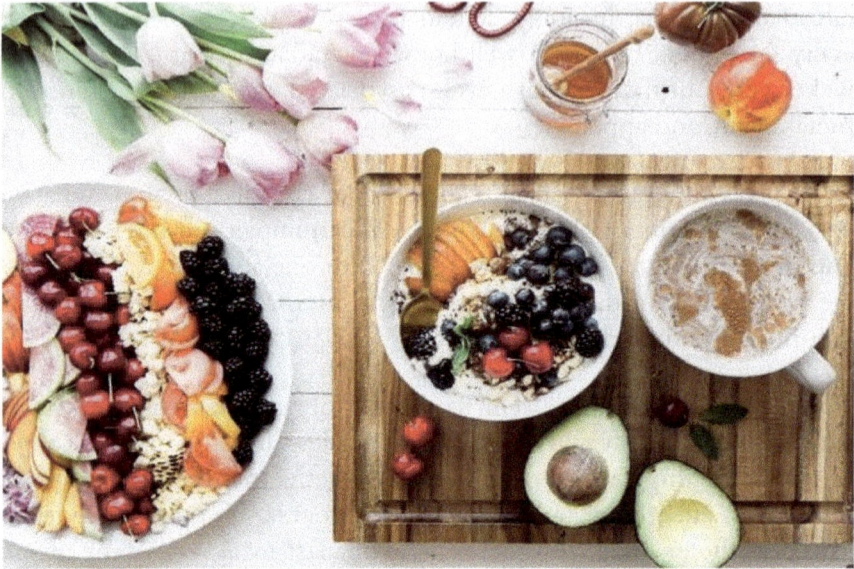

Love and Respect Your Body

How often do you look in the mirror and like your reflection? If you are like most, you probably can't remember the last time you stared at yourself in the mirror and thought how beautiful or amazing you looked. We spend an absurd amount of time disapproving of or hating our bodies because we put so much pressure on looking a certain, unrealistic way that society has conjured up. Since childhood we have had some celebrities flaunt flawless, toned bodies while others endorse one dieting method or another and magazines and the news scare us into thinking that being overweight or underweight or anything but perfect will ruin our lives.

What has hating your body done for you so far? What if, instead of cringing at your own reflection, you were able to smile and appreciate all your body has done for you? Without the body you have right now you would not be the person you are. It may feel like your body is a punishment, but when we hate how we look we are less inclined to care for ourselves the way our body needs. This neglect, over time, is what leads to poor health.

Loving and respecting your body does not mean you have to love everything about it. We all have a feature or something that we can't stand:that birthmark on your back; the way your hair frizzes after the rain; or, the way your pinky and ring finger never lay fully straight. We all have imperfections that we do not like, but it does not mean you can't accept them as part of who you are.

You may have a negative body image because of excess weight around the abdomen, or because your arms are starting to get heavy and saggy with skin. You do not have to love these things but you do have to accept and respect your body. It is only when you respect yourself that you will become more mindful of how you treat your body. How do you shift from attitudes of disgust and dissatisfaction to a state of acceptance and respect?

There are a handful of ways you can begin to respect your body, such as:

- Eat when your body gives you hunger cues.
- Move your body in a way that makes you feel good.
- Talk to yourself with more kindness.
- Show yourself compassion.
- Do not punish yourself for eating foods you like.

The problem is that most people have convinced themselves that they have to reach their weight-loss goals or look a certain way before they can begin to show their body the love and respect it deserves. What if you start now?

What would you do differently if your body looked different? Would you buy more clothes or buy more expensive clothes? Take extra time in the morning to get ready? Would you eat nourishing foods regularly? You shouldn't want your body to change before you can start loving it. Imagine how different you would feel about yourself if you start focusing on your positive traits and how good it feels to take care of yourself, instead of being obsessed with how much you despise the way you look?

How Does Food Make You Feel?

One of the best ways we can begin to respect our body is by ensuring it is getting what it needs to function. We've discussed the nutrients you need to consume so your systems run smoothly and keep you in good health. When we eat nourishing foods we feel more energized, lighter, and able to move our body with less restrictions.

Consider tracking what you eat and identifying how your body feels physically. Do you feel bloated? Lethargic? Do not focus on how you feel emotionally. We will cover that topic later in the book. For now, focus on how what you eat affects your daily physical functions.

Track your food intake and how you physically feel after eating for two weeks. Then choose three consecutive days during which you commit to eating nourishing foods. Choose to freely eat vegetables when you feel hungry. Eat a nice balance of lean meats, whole grains, and fats. Have fruit for desserts. It is important to avoid processed foods or prepackaged foods. Remember, you are only doing it for three days. During these three days again track your food consumption and how you physically feel after eating.

After the three days, compare your results and comments from the two weeks to that from the three days. Ask yourself honestly, would you rather regularly feel like you did for the two weeks or like you did for the three days? Once they experience the physical differences that result from eating nourishing foods, most people use this experience as motivation and a reminder to continue to choose foods that properly fuel their body. So many of us have simply gotten used to feeling discomfort from eating that it has become normal.

Hunger Cues

The body naturally lets us know when it needs fuel, has had enough to eat, and whether or not it actually enjoys what we are eating. The problem is, we have turned out these cues. While caregivers and parents are well-meaning, the expectation they placed on us as young children is what begins to alter our relationship with food. By the time we reach adulthood, we are completely out of touch with our body's natural cue. This leads to us misinterpreting the cues and eating when we aren't hungry.

Respecting our body begins with trusting that it tells us what it needs when it needs it. Regularly check in with your body throughout the day and ask how hungry you are. Use the hunger-fullness scale below to help determine where your hunger falls. Items one to five focus on hunger while items five to ten measure your fullness once you start eating.

1. You are starving. You may feel dizzy, nauseous, have hunger pains, or have a headache because of how hungry you are.

2. You are extremely hungry. You may be experiencing headaches, mood swings, and trouble focusing. Your stomach will be growling and you begin to feel anxious about eating.

3. You are very hungry and need to eat. You may notice you are thinking about food more frequently, your stomach is rumbling, and you may begin to feel slightly anxious about needing to eat.

4. You feel hungry and should eat soon. You might begin to notice your stomach rumbling.

5. You are beginning to feel hungry.

6. You are not full yet. You may begin to feel slightly full but can still eat a little more.

7. You can stop eating. You are feeling satisfied with how much you have eaten.

8. You have eaten a little too much. You may feel a little uncomfortable from overeating.

9. You are full. You feel stuffed, your stomach may be protruding out, and you feel incredibly uncomfortable. Your clothes feel tighter and you may even feel a little nauseous.

10. You are painfully full. You feel physically sick, lethargic, and may only be focusing on how uncomfortable you feel from eating too much.

When using this scale, you want to begin eating when you are around four or three and stop eating when you are around seven. It is important that you check in with your hunger as you eat, so you avoid overeating.

Chapter 4:

Start Small

Habits form when we are consistent and being consistent is easier when we put our full focus on one small change at a time. Now that you have a clear understanding of what your body needs, it is time to start thinking about how you can better provide it with the nourishment it requires. Many people think that creating a habit requires an excessive amount of effort. At the beginning it will take more will-power and thought, however once you adjust to the new routine your brain will automatically begin to work with you to make the new routine as effortless as possible. Over time you will simply do the actions without having to fight with yourself.

When it comes to forming a habit, understand that you want to start with the easiest possible change. Many people make the mistake of trying to make too many changes or force one big change at the beginning. This often leads to disappointment and giving up altogether. It is the smallest changes that will build your momentum. By consistently performing the same small action, you will be surprised by how much you change in a short period of time.

Compounding Eating Habits

Starting with a single small change instead of one massive commitment or multiple changes will ensure you stick with a new way of eating for the long term. Just as interest can compound on the money in your savings account, so do the results you experience from consistently implementing one small change at a time.

Many fail to lose weight and stay on track with healthier living because they have a rush of motivation and eagerness in the first few days of a new diet or exercise routine, and then that motivation falters. Temptation gets the best of them and everything and anything is better than lacing up running shoes and breaking a sweat.

Life happens. It is understandable why eating the way we should or moving more gets pushed to the back burner. What matters most is what you do most often. You are not going to gain 10 pounds overnight from enjoying a slice of birthday cake or having dessert after dinner. You also are not going to lose 10 pounds overnight by eating one salad. It is what we do consistently that will get us results. We do have control over what those results will be, however.

Habit Stacking

The more effortless it is to implement the change the more likely you are to stick with it. Additionally, the easier the change appears to be the more likely you are to exceed your expectations. The smallest change is essential because it is so small there will be little resistance to performing the action. For example, which are you more likely to do:

- Go for a 20 minute run five times a week.

- Put your shoes on and walk around the block once every morning.

The second one is more appealing because it takes less effort and little commitment. But, what happens when you've been walking around the block for two or three weeks? You begin to tell yourself to circle around two blocks. Then three. You will continue to add distance and speed until you are easily running 20 minutes, five times a week. On the other hand, if you try to start out with the first option, especially when you haven't run in a while, you will start running and 30 seconds or a minute into your run you will be huffing and puffing and having to stop. You turn around and head back home defeated. It is highly unlikely you will attempt that 20 minute run again.

The best approach to making a new habit stick is to sneak it into a routine you already do daily. For example, say you want to start by drinking more water throughout the day, think about your routines and identify how you can add drinking a glass of water into one of them. Maybe you could have a glass of water sitting next to your bed and as soon as you get up you reach for that cup and drink it before you reach for your phone or turn on your light. Maybe in the car on your commute to work you set a coffee cup of water in your cup holder instead of your typical cup of joe. The goal is to seamlessly slip the new habit into your routine so it doesn't disrupt what you are already doing. This allows you to quickly attach a trigger to perform the new habit.

To help identify and plug in your new habits, complete one of the sentences below:

After (CURRENT HABIT), I will (NEW HABIT).

or

Before (CURRENT HABIT), I will (NEW HABIT).

Some examples of how this would look:

- After I start my morning coffee, I will meditate for two minutes.

- Before I sit down at my desk, I will fill my water bottle.

- After I drop the kids off at school, I will walk around the building one time.

- Before I begin to eat, I will pause to appreciate the food.

- After I put the kids to bed, I will read for 10 minutes.

- Before I get into bed, I will prepare my gym bag for the morning.

- After I clean up from dinner, I will pack my lunch for the next day.

Once you have established how to fit in one new habit, you can begin to stack others on top. For example, if you start with: After I start my morning coffee, I will meditate for two minutes. You can add:

- After I meditate for two minutes, I will stretch for five minutes,

- After I stretch for five minutes, I will drink a glass of water.

- After I drink a glass of water, I will eat a banana.

Consider also where you can begin to set up a new habit to perform later in an already established routine. For example, you want to make journaling a habit in the evening before you go to bed. You can place the journal on your pillow after you make your bed. By placing it on your pillow you have to physically move it before you go to sleep which will be the reminder you need to open it up and write in it.

Remember, the cue to start the habits is essential. Do not just stick to a new habit where you want it to fit. Sometimes we need to carefully examine our already established routine to ensure we can commit to the habit for the long term. For example, you may want to stack a habit of working out into your morning routine. But your mornings are already chaotic and getting up any earlier would require far more effort then you are willing to commit. No matter where you try to squeeze this habit into your morning it will not stick. You can either find another time during the day to make it work or you can begin creating a habit stack that will lead to making your mornings less chaotic and open up time to do a work out.

Four Core Habits to Build On

You already know these habits but are you implementing them? So many know they are supposed to drink more water and eat their veggies but they fail to do these small actions. The main reason people do not stick to what they should be doing is that they overcomplicate it. This section simplifies how to take action and stick with the simple habits that are essential for weight loss.

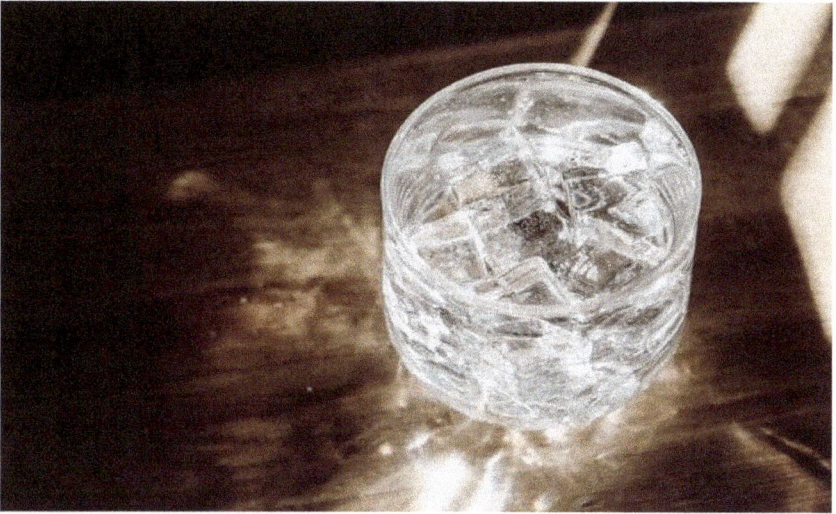

Drink More Water

Adding more cups of H_2O to your day can help you manage or lose weight. Many confuse thirst with hunger, which means we tend to eat and consume unnecessary calories when we need to be hydrated. Drinking more water aids in weight loss in a few key ways:

- Drinking water suppresses the appetite.

- Drinking cold water boosts metabolism because the body needs to use extra energy to warm the water before it uses it (Boschmann et al., 2003). This also means you burn more calories while at rest.

- The body needs a sufficient water supply to assist in fat metabolism.

- Drinking more water helps reduce the number of calorie drinks you consume.

Though we almost always have access to water and can easily carry it with us, very few adults drink enough water to keep their body functioning properly.

There are some simple ways you can begin to increase your water consumption slowly every day. First, track how much water you are actually drinking during the day. Do not try to increase your water intake yet. Instead, go through your days as you normally do and note when and how much water you drink. Track your daily water intake for two weeks; this establishes a starting point for increasing your water intake. Once you have your starting point, calculate how much water you should be consuming each day (covered in the previous chapter). After establishing your water intake goal, begin to add eight ounces more a day. Some ways you can do this include:

- Keep a glass of water next to your bed. As soon as you wake up in the morning, drink the water.

- Drink a glass of water before you eat your meals.

- Drink a glass of water as soon as you get to work.

- Take a sip of water before you reach for a snack when hungry. Wait and see if your hunger diminishes.

- If you enjoy sweet beverages, alternate them with water. Once you finish 8-ounces of water, drink a beverage of your choice of equal size (8-ounces). Continue to alternate through the day.

- Keep a bottle of water in your car, in your office, or at your work station.

- Fill a reusable bottle to carry with you when you have to run errands. If you already have it accessible when you are out of the house you are more likely to drink it.

- Eat more fruit and vegetables with high-water content.

- Soups, stews, and smoothies can also help you add a little extra water into your diet.

- Drink a glass of water each time you brush your teeth.

Look at your daily routine and identify just one consistent time of day where you can sneak in a glass of water. After a week or two of adding eight extra ounces, add another eight. Continue adding eight ounces at a time until you have reached your water goal. You can flavor your water with fruits and vegetables to keep it more interesting and help you stick with and maintain your new water habits.

Keep in mind, there are some days you should drink extra water. When the weather is hot or humid it is important to drink more water to avoid dehydrations. On days you are more physically active you should drink more water to help the muscles function properly and replace water lost to sweat or perspiration.

Eat More Vegetables

The next healthy habit you want to focus on is to increase your vegetable intake. Vegetables can be added to nearly any dish, yet a majority of us struggle to get in even one daily serving of vegetables. Many people avoid eating vegetables because they think it takes too much extra time to clean, chop, and cook them. Plus, if you haven't found vegetables you enjoy eating, it can be hard to eat more because you do not know what you like or how to cook them in a way that you like.

Vegetables are essential for eating a well-balanced diet. They also provide the body with a majority of the vitamins, minerals, and other nutrients needed for optimal health. There are five key ways that eating more vegetables will help you lose weight:

- Most vegetables are high in fiber and water which help you feel full faster.

- Vegetables have fewer calories, meaning you get to eat them freely without worrying about packing on extra pounds.

- When you combine vegetables with lean protein and healthy fats you feel more satisfied after eating.

- When you eat enough vegetables throughout the day you will feel more energized so you are able to get more done and will burn more calories without hitting an afternoon slump or feeling completely drained by the end of the day.

- Vegetables can help eliminate or decrease sugar cravings, so you do not consume excess calories.

Once again, you want to know where you are starting, so for two week track what you eat. It is important to stick with your normal eating patterns so you get an honest look at what you eat. Many people are unaware of how few vegetables they eat. They often think they are eating significantly more than they do, you might surprise yourself. Even if you go days without eating vegetables, that is OK. This is not about shaming you into eating better, it is about guiding you to make necessary changes for a healthier life.

To start incorporating more vegetables, start with just a half cup, one day a week. If you notice through your tracking you are already getting a serving of vegetables daily then choose one day to start increasing your consumption by just a half cup at a time. A half a cup does not look or feel like a lot. You may be thinking already, *A half a cup is not going to change anything.* Which is true. If you stop at half a cup.

Remember, we are compounding these habits. A half cup is easy to accomplish but—in the beginning—it is just as easy not to do it. Once you add a half a cup one day a week you will add to it each week.

You can add the half cup each week one of two ways. You can continue to add another half cup on the same day each week, or you can add a half cup to another day in the week. Continue to add a half cup each week until you have reached either three cups at least one day a week or a half a cup of vegetables everyday of the week. Stick with this pattern for at least two weeks then begin adding half cups again until you are eating three cups of vegetables every day.

To make the process easier consider the following tips on how to increase your veggie consumption.

- Experiment with veggie noodles or veggie rice (cauliflower rice). You do not have to replace your traditional noodles or white rice completely with veggie noodles or cauliflower rice. To start, simply replace a portion of the pasta you would eat during your meal with vegetable noodles: zucchini noodles, sliced eggplant for lasagna noodles, and shredded carrots. Do the same with any rice dishes.

- You can also just add steamed or roasted vegetables into your pasta dishes. Toss broccoli, brussels sprouts, zucchini, and spinach in with your pasta noodles.

- Use lettuce wraps and vegetable buns instead of white tortillas and bread. Portobello mushroom caps make great buns for burgers.

- Sneak vegetables into sauces and smoothies. Baby spinach, carrots, and beets are sweeter vegetables that blend nicely in fruit smoothies.

- Snack on raw vegetables sticks paired with a dip or spread. Celery with cream cheese or peanut butter, carrot sticks with peanut butter, mini bell peppers with tuna salad or cucumber slices with hummus are all filling and satisfying snacks that you can grab in between meals.

- Add extra vegetables into soups and stews. You can also incorporate various vegetables like eggplant, zucchini, peppers, and onions into recipes like chili and omelets. Mushrooms can be added to nearly any meat recipe including meatloaf and tacos.

- Add vegetables to your sandwiches, wraps, and burgers. You can also top your handheld meals with lettuce, tomatoes, and onions but mix it up and add some sauteed peppers, pickled onions, mushrooms, or cabbage slaw.

- Top your pizza with vegetables.

As you can see, there are plenty of ways to incorporate vegetables into all your meals and snacks throughout the day. With so many options, you will find that reaching your three cups a day goals will be accomplished in no time.

Include More Whole Grains

When people think of adding in whole grains most immediately think of brown rice, or whole wheat pasta and bread. These are great starting points, but whole grains consist of more than just flour and pasta. Other whole grains you can try include:

- oats
- quinoa
- buckwheat
- millet
- wild rice
- dark rye
- bulgur
- spelt

Whole grains contain various nutrients that maintain a healthy lifestyle and weight. The body processes whole grains differently than it does refined grains, which is why they are ideal for helping you reach your weight loss goals. Whole grains promote weight loss because:

- They reduce the number of calories the body stores.

- They boost metabolism and can increase your resting metabolic rate. This results in the body burning more calories throughout the day.

- Eating whole grains can help you burn an extra 100 calories a day. This is the same number of calories you would burn if you walked at a moderate pace for 30 minutes.

- Many whole-grains contain plenty of fiber which helps you feel full for longer.

When adding more whole grains into your diet it is important to keep the suggested servings size in mind. This is not about restricting how much you eat, it is about understanding how much is enough to fuel the body effectively without overconsuming storing excesses as fat.

Many neglect serving sizes when eating or portioning a plate of food, so it can be a huge adjustment for most who are used to eating big bowls of pasta and rice. For example, a serving of whole wheat bread is one slice. A serving of whole-wheat pasta is around half a cup.

There are many ways you can increase your whole-grain intake.

- Do not skip breakfast. Try eating a serving of oats or a slice of whole-grain toast with avocado and sliced hard boiled egg.

- Combine your whole wheat with your refined grains. Start by adding a quarter cup of whole-grain pasta then, slowly bump up how much whole-grain pasta you add by a quarter cup each time you make a pasta or rice dish.

- Use whole grains as a snack, such as plain popcorn, or whole wheat crackers with nut butter.

- Experiment with a new grain every month.

One thing to be aware of when you begin shopping for whole grains is to always double-check the labels. Do not get fooled by labels that state the product is 'multigrain' or consists of "seven grains." These products often contain more refined grains than whole grains. When reading the labels be sure that whole wheat or another whole grain is listed within the first five ingredients. This tells you that the whole grain is a primary ingredient. The further down an ingredient is listed, the smaller its amount in the product.

Choose More Lean Proteins

Lean protein does not refer to just animal meat. Eggs, dairy, nuts, legumes, spinach, and whole grains all contain adequate amounts of protein. You probably eat plenty of meat products now, this habit is about adding lean sources over poor-quality protein such as processed meats or fat-laden cuts of beef and pork.

When choosing meats choose grass-fed and wild-range options as these contain more nutrients. Focus on choosing leaner cuts of meat. A sirloin steak will often be larger in portion size but will have fewer calories than a fuller or fatty cut of meat like a T-bone steak.

As we discussed in the previous chapter, protein is an essential nutrient the body needs. It is also an important component to eating a well-balanced diet to support weight loss. Lean proteins help boost weight loss in a number of ways, which include:

- Eating lean protein helps reduce the risk of overeating because it helps you feel full and satisfied.

- Lean protein is essential for building muscles. Muscle helps burn more calories.

- The body needs to use more energy to digest protein which results in using more calories during the digestion process.

- When we eat protein it triggers the body to stop producing ghrelin, the hunger hormone.

Keep in mind that, as with most foods, just consuming more protein is not going to lead to weight loss. You should be eating enough protein to help provide the body with what it needs. As a general rule, you should try to eat 0.4 grams of protein for every pound of body weight (Frey, 2021). If you weigh 180 pounds that means you should be eating 72 grams of protein a day, or 2.5 ounces.

Some ways to begin adding more lean protein to your diet include:

- Consume omega-rich fish, like salmon, once a week.

- Add a protein source to your breakfast such as eggs or black beans. Eating eggs in the morning has shown to help reduce appetite throughout the morning, which leads to less snacking (Spritzler, 2021).

- Go with a plant-based recipe once a week. Instead of traditional chili made from ground meat, go with a meatless chili made with black and kidney beans.

- Snack on nuts, cheese, cottage cheese, Greek yogurt, and nut butter spread on whole-grain bread or with apple slices.

- Add almonds or other nuts to salads, yogurt, or oats.

You should aim to include one small portion of protein with every meal. Creating a meal plan is an effective way to ensure that you are getting the right balance of protein every day. With this approach you start by planning out one meal a week, for example plan out all your lunches for the week. Once you have gotten used to planning and preparing one meal, plan another, until you naturally create a menu for all your meals and snacks each week.

It is important to notice that each of these habits emphasizes 'more.' Drink more water, eat more greens, by focusing on the 'more' you trick the mind to focus on what you are getting more of rather than focusing on what you are cutting back on. If you phrase these changes differently and start off by saying, "Drink less soda," you immediately think you are depriving the body. Always think in terms of how much more nutritious food and drink you are consuming instead of thinking about the other stuff you are eating less of.

Chapter 5:

Habits Holding You Back

Now that you have your four habits to start with it is time to take a look into the current habits you may be exhibiting. There are several habits, and not all have to do with what you eat, that will hinder your weight loss efforts. To make the necessary changes we need to first clarify what is keeping us from our goals. By identifying the poor eating and lifestyle habits we participate in we can begin to combat them with effective tools and strategies.

Review each of these habits carefully. You may not think that you engage in certain habits, but after learning more about them, you'll find that you are guilty of more than one item on this list. Do not feel mad if you have one or all of these habits; all habits can be changed or eliminated. However, we can't change the things we do not admit we are doing.

Mindless Snacking

When we eat mindlessly, we tend to eat when we are not hungry. We either reach for food because it is in sight or we are not engaged fully during the eating process. Mindless eating occurs when we eat more than we intend to because we are not paying attention to the cues from our body.

There are many things internally and externally that can cause us to shift our focus away from eating. Emotions and thoughts can play a major role in causing you to mindlessly eat. Environmental factors like the television, who you are with, and whether you are sitting and eating or on the go as you eat can contribute to being unaware of how much you are eating.

Practicing mindful eating is the best way to remain present and tuned into your body as you eat. Being aware of what factors may contribute to mindless eating is also essential, but you must come up with a plan to combat these factors. For instance, you can avoid eating out of bags or containers and instead have a small bowl of snacks while you watch television.

Make it a priority to sit and eat. We are more likely to overeat throughout the day if we are constantly reaching for things that we can "grab and go" with. Sitting and enjoying your meal will help you remain present in the entire eating experience. This also provides you the opportunity to check-in with your hunger cues to ensure that you aren't over eating.

Grazing

How often do you notice reaching for a bag of chips or picking up another piece of candy from the dish on your desk or kitchen counter? You may or may not notice how much you snack throughout the day which only hinders any weight loss efforts.

Grazing like this is often caused by boredom, but can also be a habitual action. Stepping into your office may trigger you to head straight for the candy dish that is always available. Walking into your own kitchen may trigger the same reaction. Grazing may also be an eating pattern you developed as you aged. Since most people do not sit down to eat each of their meals, they have gotten into the habit of just grabbing food when it is accessible.

The best way to address this eating habit is to remove temptation or, at least, make snacks that are easy to grab far less accessible. Sometimes just putting food out of sight can help those with grazing tendencies to stop, others need to put food on the highest counter they can or in a completely different room so they have to move a chair or go down a flight of stairs to reach it.

Instead of having food within reach, have a bottle of water nearby. When you feel a hunger pang reach for your water rather than a snack. If drinking water doesn't eliminate your hunger then have a snack that consists of protein, fat, and fiber like apple slices or celery sticks with nut butter.

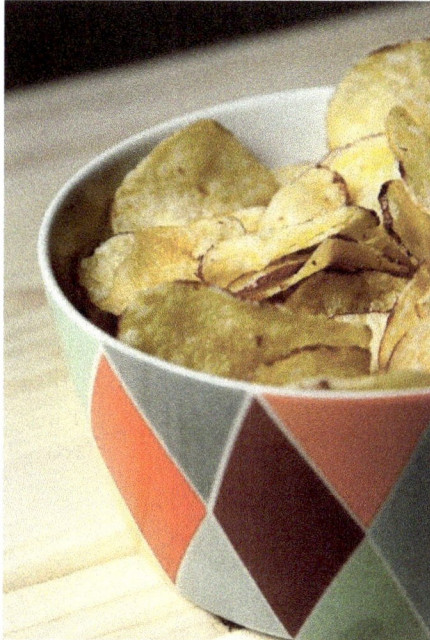

Distracted Eating

When we are distracted, we lose track of how much we are eating. How often have you sat down to watch a television show and gone through an entire bag of popcorn or chips? How many times have you started munching on crackers or told yourself you would just have a cookie or two while you scroll your social accounts, only to reach down to an empty packaging sleeve? When we engage in distracted eating, while engaged in a mindless activity like these, we tend to overeat because we are multitasking, eating being one of the tasks. It is impossible for our brains to focus fully on more than one task at a time. Trying to do something else while we eat causes our brain to focus on the other activity which means we do not realize how much we are eating.

Distracted eating can also have the opposite effect on how much we eat. How many times have you missed your lunch break because you were busy with a work task? If we are engaging in an activity that requires more cognitive effort, we often ignore our hunger cues and any food in front of us. We are still multitasking but the other activity we are doing requires us to not only focus more intently on what we are doing but often requires us to physically move more, such as responding to an email or finishing up a work report.

Distracted eating is common when you do not stick to a consistent eating schedule. If needed, set an alarm to go off every two to three hours to remind you it is time to eat. When the alarm goes off, turn off the electronics and sit down to eat. Also, consider having your snacks portioned out to eliminate overeating in case you do get caught up in another activity.

Eating Too Quickly

When we eat too fast we tend to consume more food in a short amount of time without giving our body time to react. It takes our body around 20 minutes for communication between the brain and gut to come to an agreement on when we have had enough to eat. You can over consume a significant amount of food and feel sick, sluggish, and uncomfortable for hours after your meal.

We tend to eat until we feel full. When we combine this with eating fast, we are often left distended to the point where it is hard to move and stand. We need to recognize when we are rushing through our meals and slow down.

Before you begin to eat, incorporate some mindful eating techniques. Take a few moments to enjoy how your food looks and smells. When you take your first bite, focus on how the food tastes and the textures as you chew. When you swallow, pause before you take another bite. Imagine the food traveling down to your stomach.

As you eat, set your utensils down between bites. This will help you slow down because you aren't focusing on getting more food on your fork or spoon and can take your time with each bite. You do not have to give every bite your full attention, but be sure to check in with yourself after every three or four bites.

Remember to measure your fullness and satisfaction. When you begin to feel full, stop eating. When you begin to notice you aren't enjoying what you are eating, stop eating. Our satisfaction tends to diminish significantly after the second bite, but we get into the habit of trying to recreate the enjoyment we had with the first bite. You may notice this especially with desserts or sweets. That first bite you take is fully satisfying. You even pause without thinking to savor the taste. You take another bite and are still feeling the pleasure from the first bite. By the third bite, you start thinking that chocolate cake is too rich or too sweet, but you have that recent memory of how blissful it was just a few bites ago. Many of us continue to eat what we initially enjoyed because we need to continue to enjoy it. This often results in overeating and making ourselves sick. Once you notice you aren't enjoying what you ate as much, allow yourself to stop.

Skipping Meals

When we skip meals we are more prone to binge or overeat later in the day. We are all guilty of forgetting to eat with a busy schedule and a majority of people skip their first meal of the day. However, of all the meals we shouldn't miss, breakfast is the most important.

Eating breakfast helps kick our metabolism in gear. Those who eat breakfast are less likely to struggle with cravings. Breakfast is crucial for maintaining a healthy weight. Eating breakfast also helps you regulate your eating schedule. It allows you to reset your internal clock and helps sync your systems back to their natural mode of operation.

You may not feel hungry in the morning and grabbing a cup of coffee and heading out the door seems much easier than cooking up something at the start of your day. Eating something small like a piece of fruit before you drink your morning coffee can help suppress your appetite.

You do not want to force yourself to eat a big meal if you are not hungry. However, you do want to have something on hand when you begin to feel the first signs of hunger, which will usually start to occur one to three hours after you wake. Prepare some overnight oats or a breakfast sandwich that you can grab and take with you when hunger does arise.

Shopping When Hungry

How often have you gone to the grocery store on an empty stomach and suddenly everything looks good or you end up buying way too much food because you can't decide on what you want to eat? Our eyes are much bigger than our stomach and our reason and logical skills are slightly impaired when we are hungry. This is why you notice you spend much more at the store when you are hungry, even if you have a list.

It is always best to have a light snack with you if you know you are going to be running errands for a good portion of the day. Try to plan your shopping trips after you eat. Always stick to a list. While this may not help if you are hungry, shopping from a list can minimize how much extra food you might place in your cart. Additionally, if you know you will be tempted to stop at a fast food place before or after your shopping trip because you are hungry, have another route planned out so you can avoid driving past these establishments, if possible.

Takeout and Processed Foods Make Up A Majority of Your Diet

Many people immediately think that they need to cut back on sugar items and snack foods to help lose weight. So they cut these foods out but are disappointed when the weight doesn't start coming off. For most, it is not the fact that they are eating a lot of sweets or snacks but that they are eating unbalanced meals that include a lot of processed and prepackaged food that is the problem.

How often do you resort to throwing a premade item in the microwave for breakfast and lunch? How many of your dinner foods come from a box? Most people consume an excessive amount of processed foods which adds a lot of calories to your day and few nutrients.

Consuming processed foods like pre-made meals and side dishes will hinder your weight loss efforts. These foods do not include many plant based sources, so we are not getting the proper nutrients our body needs. Even things like frozen vegetable dishes that are in a sauce are often precooked and have their nutrients stripped during the process.

If we are lacking the nutrients essential for our body to function we will continue to feel hungry. Have you ever noticed that when you eat take-out food, like Chinese food, you can eat until you are so stuffed you feel sick but then 20 minutes later you are still hungry? This is because we are not getting the sufficient nutrients we need from our meals.

Take an honest look at what you eat during a typical day and week. Notice when you are more likely to turn to something quick and easy to make. Then, begin to create a meal plan that works with your schedule. Not many of us have the time or energy to make a home cooked meal every night. However, you can take some time once or twice a week to prepare meals that you can easily freeze and reheat later. The goal is to create meals that take little time to get on the table while incorporating foods that will help fill you up and provide the right balance of nutrients.

Sugar

Do not drink your carbs or calories. Many sugar-filled drinks are absurdly high in calories and lack any beneficial nutrients. Many people who struggle with weight loss ignore what they drink when it comes to the overall diet. Since these drinks contain a high number of calories we are supplying the body with excess fuel it can't use, so it has to be stored as fat.

Sugar is a hard item to eliminate from our diet because of how the brain reacts to consuming it. Processed sugar, like the white table sugar you probably have in your pantry, triggers the brain's reward system. This is why so many of us crave sweets. Additionally, we will crave sugar when under stress because of the body's natural flight or flight defense mechanism (which will be discussed later in the book). This does not mean you cannot become more aware of how much sugar you consume throughout the day and begin to change certain drinks or foods for others.

You have been told to swap out your sugary beverages for water and in the last chapter we discussed various ways to drink more water. But, for many, water doesn't give them the same satisfaction as flavored drinks. You can try to add more flavor to your water by adding fruit like strawberries, raspberries, watermelon, or kiwi to a pitcher of water. You can also make drinks like lemonade but use honey to sweeten it instead of white table sugar.

Also, when you get sweet cravings, reach for a piece of fruit. The fruit is naturally sweet and will provide you with essential vitamins that can help combat sugar cravings. Additionally, recognize that your sugar cravings can be due to stress, lack of sleep, or other emotional needs. Do not immediately cave in to your sugar cravings. Instead, get into the habit of asking yourself what your body is actually telling you it needs when you have a craving for sugar or sugary drinks and food.

Caffeine

Some people recommend drinking a cup of balck coffee to help boost weight loss, but this advice can be misleading. While drinking a cup of black coffee in the morning might make you feel a little more energized, it often causes negative effects later in the day. Caffeine can interfere with sleep, especially when you consume it later in the day. It can also increase sugar cravings because consuming too much caffeine can elevate cortisol levels in the body.

While you do not have to give up your cup of coffee in the morning, you should stick with only a cup or two to the early half of your day. Set a cut-off time for your last cup of coffee so it doesn't interfere with your sleep. If you are feeling like you need a boost of energy, which caffeine would typically supply, try going for a brisk walk or splashing cold water on your face.

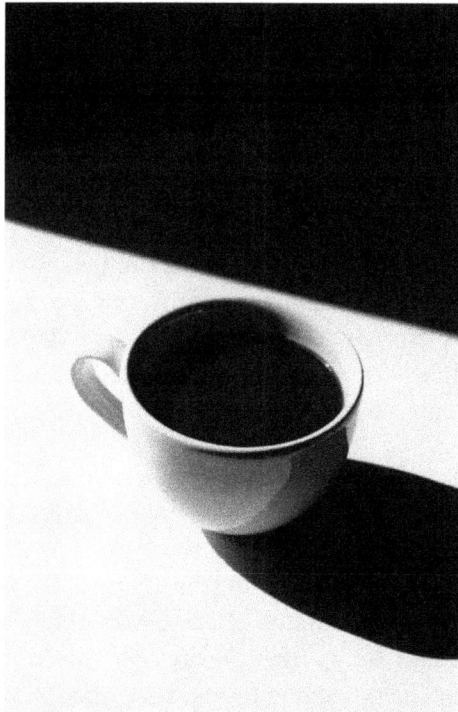

Not Prioritizing Sleep

There is a strong correlation between sleep and eating habits. Too little sleep often results in food choices that hinder weight loss. Since we tend to crave sugary foods when we are tired, we will reach for them first.

Also, sleep plays an integral rule in maintaining our circadian rhythms (as discussed in Chapter 3). If we skip on sleep, we throw off our internal clock and feel hungry when our metabolism is at its lowest and kick on the digestive process when we should be resting.

Additionally, when we do not get enough sleep, the hormones that control hunger and fullness become unbalanced. The body produces more ghrelin, which is our hunger hormone, and is slow to release leptin, the hormone which suppresses our hunger. We feel more hungry when we are tired and we need to consume more food before feeling satiated.

It is vital that you begin to make sleep a priority if you want to lose weight and keep it off. Begin by setting a regular bedtime. Have an evening routine that promotes sleep. Incorporate calming activities like meditation, journaling, and reading that will help you feel sleepy.

Be sure your sleep environment also encourages a good night's sleep. Keep electronics off, this might mean putting your phone in another room or far away from your bed. If necessary wear a sleep mask to block out any light as you sleep. Keep the temperature of your room to around 68°F. Be sure your bedroom has proper air circulation.

Also, be mindful of what you eat and when your last meal is. Certain foods may cause you to remain awake such as simple carbohydrates or spicy foods. You also want to ensure that your last meal is at least two hours before bed. If you are feeling hungry before bed, stick to light foods like Greek yogurt, cottage cheese, or a slice of turkey. Be sure not to drink too many fluids right before bed so you do not wake up in the middle of your sleep needing to get out of bed.

You may need to make a few adjustments to your sleep environment and evening activities to ensure that you are getting the quality sleep you need. If you find that you still struggle with falling asleep or staying asleep it is encouraged that you speak to your doctor. Poor sleep can be an indication of serious conditions that you should address sooner rather than later.

Chapter 6:

Addressing Emotional Eating

We are all guilty of feeding our emotions at one time or another. For some, emotional eating has become a normal way of eating and often leads to overeating. Emotional eating is one of the most common eating habits that hinders weight loss efforts.

Many of us feel completely justified to treat ourselves with favorite foods when dealing with difficult emotions. This is another habit that could have been encouraged through childhood and your teenage years. How often did you reach for a tub of ice cream after a break up? Did your mom or grandmother bake you a batch of homemade cookies when you achieved something? How often did you witness your parents sneak a few pieces of candy after a stressful day of work? Unknowingly, you may be feeding your emotions more often than you realize.

You need to learn how to identify triggers of emotional eating. Once you know what emotions or situations trigger your urge to eat, we can come up with an effective plan to manage our emotions and reactions to them better.

Implementing better coping mechanisms is not just essential for weight loss. properly managing emotions and allowing yourself to feel what you are feeling without numbing them or stuffing them down will lead to improved mental health.

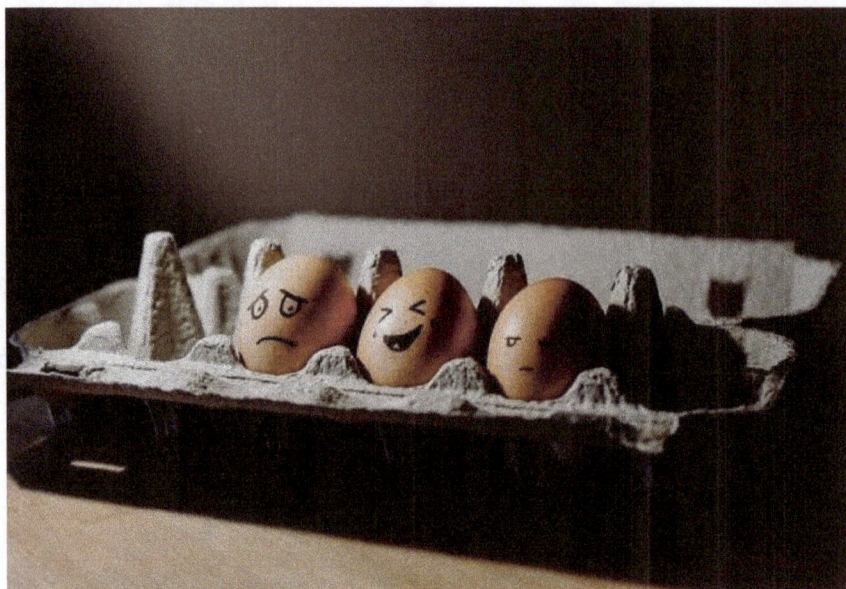

Why We Eat With Our Emotions

Everyone has taken part in emotional eating at some point in their life and doing it every once in a while is harmless. However, constantly turning to food for comfort or an escape from feeling certain emotions leads to long-term problems.

When you constantly pick up your favorite pint of ice cream or a milkshake from you favorite fast-food place when you've had a bad day, failed a test, or had a fight with your partner, these once-in-a-while occasions begin to train your brain to signal for these foods every times you encounter an upsetting emotion.

We are also hardwired to crave certain foods when we experience certain emotions. Unfortunately, some of the natural biological responses our brain has to things like stress are outdated. Our bodies still operate like our ancestors' did when fearing for their life because of a predator. When we experience certain emotions, our brains do not differentiate between what is a real and serious threat and what is just an overreaction or responding to an upsetting, but not life-threatening, situation.

Have you noticed that when you feel a certain way you tend to crave a specific type of food? For many, these cravings tend to focus on sweets and carbohydrates. These foods supply our body with fuel and if you were in a situation where you needed to fight or run for your life, your body would rely on the instant and extra energy these foods provide. Since we rarely find ourselves in life-threatening situations, we need to learn how to identify these cravings and then provide the body with what it needs.

Binge Eating

Emotional eating is one of the most common factors that lead to binge eating. Binge eating occurs when we consume a substantial amount of food in a very short period of time. While we are guilty of binging once in a while, for instance at a holiday gathering, it is a habit that can lead to more serious, disordered eating conditions.

Binge eating is a concern when it interferes with our daily living. Most who struggle with a binge eating disorder feel out of control around food. They tend to segregate themselves so others will not discover their poor eating habits. After a binging episode, the binger experiences shame, guilt, and resentment. These feelings only fuel the next episode and you find yourself in a negative feedback loop unable to break free.

The biggest issue with binge eating occurs after the binge. The shame and guilt one feels after binging is unbearable at times. This promotes a negative mindset that keeps the binger trapped in their condition.

If you feel you struggle with a binge eating disorder it is advised that you share your concerns with your healthcare provider. They can help you find additional help to address the internal conflicts you are struggling with. Do not feel ashamed if this is the case. Binge eating disorder is one of the most common eating disorders reported. You are not alone in your struggle and should not feel ashamed or embarrassed about admitting to your eating habits. Many of us need additional help to work through the years of disordered eating we have been living through.

Identifying Triggers

While our emotions are what give us the final push to eat, there are certain places, people, thoughts, or experiences that often cause the emotions that drive our urge to eat. It is crucial to start uncovering what these triggers are so you can find better coping mechanisms or create a plan on how to avoid or overcome these triggers.

To learn your triggers you need to track your eating habits. Carry around a notebook, journal, or keep a note on your phone to rack every time you eat or drink throughout the day. Be sure to include:

- The time you ate.

- What you ate.

- How you felt while you ate.

- What you were doing before you ate.

- Where you ate. Be specific. Do not just write "at home" write "while sitting on the couch" or "standing at the kitchen counter."

- Who you were with.

- What else you were doing while you ate.

- How you felt after eating.

All these observations will help you uncover the patterns of your emotional eating.

You may notice that you tend to eat more in the evening after a stressful day at work. In this case you would want to incorporate some relaxing methods into your evening routine. You might find that you overeat when you are around certain people, maybe they make you feel uncomfortable or you are trying to avoid joining the conversation because you are shy. You can either avoid hanging out with these individuals or encourage your group of friends to do another activity that doesn't involve food.

Once you uncover a pattern, you can begin to incorporate more effective coping mechanisms. As you become more aware of the influences of your emotions on your eating behaviors, you will find that it is easier to combat urges to eat in any situation.

Emotional Hunger Versus Physical Hunger

One of the reasons we tend to eat with our emotions is because we misread our emotional and physical hunger cues. To help uncover your triggers for emotional eating it helps to understand the different cues your body sends out to let you know what it needs.

With emotional hunger you are likely to experience:

- Extreme hunger very suddenly.

- Cravings for specific foods.

- A lack of control once you start eating and unable to recognize your fullness.

- Shame, guilt, or other negative feelings after you eat.

With physical hunger you will experience:

- Hunger that increases in intensity slowly.

- A desire to eat a variety of foods.

- The ability to recognize your fullness and know it is time to stop eating.

- No negative feelings after eating.

You may not be able to interpret these cues from one another when you first tune into your body. If you have struggled with emotional eating for a long time, then you can easily misunderstand both emotional and physical hunger cues. This is why it is recommended to check in with yourself and ask if there is anything else your hunger might be telling you.

One of the best ways to begin addressing emotional eating is to stick to a regular eating schedule. When you begin to eat at regular times you will be able to identify your emotional hunger from your physical hunger more easily. Try to space out your main meals every three to four hours and allow yourself to have a light snack in between meals that will hold you over until your next meal. This schedule is not meant to control your hunger: When you are feeling hungry, eat. Just be sure you have checked with your body to identify if it may be needing something other than food.

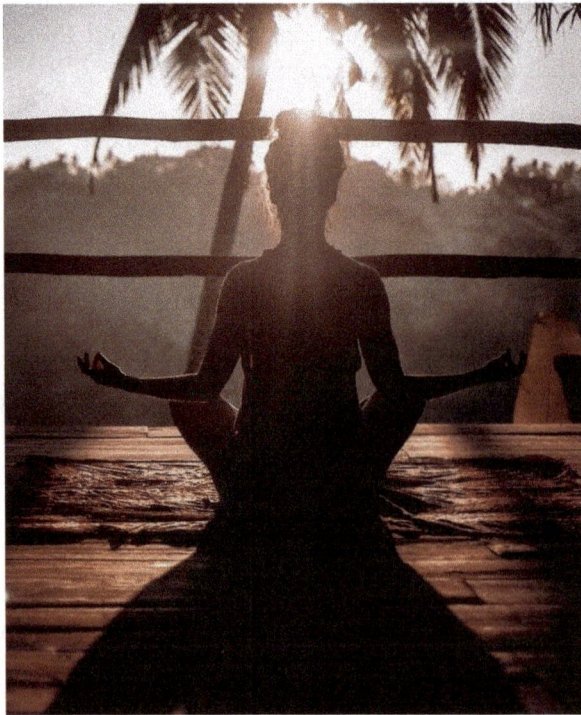

Effective Coping Mechanisms

While food is never the best option to help you cope with your feelings, you can find alternative food choices that help you feel more comforted. Instead of choosing a pint of ice cream, opt for a cup of Greek yogurt with fresh fruit or some sorbet. By switching up your food choices to help with your emotional discomfort you begin to retrain your brain to look at these better-for-you foods as comfort which, over time, results in consuming them more often.

It is ok to have a bad day and want to feel comfort and warmth, you can provide this to yourself by sipping on a cup of hot tea. Various teas have a soothing effect which will help you deal with your emotions in a more healthy way. You can also sip on some clear broth or sit down with a bowl of hearty soup, you know the kind your mom or grandmother used to have ready for you when it was freezing, snowing, or raining.

The best way to stop emotional eating is to deal with your emotions when they happen. So many of us try to hide our pain and hurt so quickly that, after years of avoiding the negative emotions, we have forgotten that they will not last forever. By allowing yourself to feel your emotions you begin to learn that it is okay to feel disappointed and upset. Once you learn to feel these emotions you can begin to address them in a more positive and healthy way. Some methods for remaining in control of your emotions include:

Meditate

Starting a meditation practice can be incredibly beneficial for your health. Despite the benefits, many people avoid meditation because it does take time to get into the habit of sitting still. Many feel they are "doing it wrong" or feel anxious about being still for more than 30 seconds.

A common misconception many have about meditation is that it requires you to sit for long periods of time chanting or repeating a mantra. Many people immediately say they do not have the time to do that. However, you do not need to spend hours sitting with your thoughts; you do not have to be sitting at all to meditate. You can begin a meditation practice that takes two minutes to complete. There are also meditations you can do as you move. The key to making meditation a habit is to find a practice that works for you.

When it comes to weight loss, there are several meditation techniques you can try to help combat emotional eating. Meditation has been shown to help reduce stress, which is a common trigger for emotional eating. It is also a way to help you identify negative thoughts patterns around eating and food that you can reframe. Some meditation techniques to try include:

Loving Kindness Meditation

Loving kindness meditation is beneficial for tuning into your own needs as well as learning to forgive and release disappointment from your day. During this meditation you receive and send loving messages. You can sit or lay for this practice.

Begin by focusing on your breath, do not try to control it, allow yourself to inhale and exhale naturally. As you breathe, begin to give thanks to your body that allows you to breathe in and out as you are. Think about your day. What has your body allowed you to accomplish? Give thanks for all the work it has done. Next, begin to think about what you ate and give thanks for being able to eat each of your meals. Appreciate all the times you fueled your body or kept it hydrated. You can continue the practice by sending messages of love to the people you know. When you are done, return your focus to your breath. Send out one last loving message to your body.

Breath Awareness

This meditation technique is what many think of when they hear 'meditation.' In breath awareness practice, you focus on your breath for a specific number of counts.

You inhale for a count of three to five and exhale for the same number of counts. During this proactive practice, the goal is to recognize when thoughts or external stimuli distract you from your breath. When you do notice your thoughts going elsewhere, you guide your mind back to your breath.

Breath meditation is an effective way to combat stress. It can also be practiced just before you eat so you can shut off the distracting chatter in your head to focus on enjoying your meals. When you become overwhelmed with intense emotions, stopping to focus on your breath can help calm your mind and improve your concentration. This allows you enough time to pause before you react to your emotions so you can handle them more effectively.

Breath meditation can be done anywhere and for as long as you decide. You can take a minute during your workday to sit at your desk to focus on your breathing. You can create a meditation space in your home to practice for five to thirty minutes. When first beginning this practice it is best to keep the time to just two or three minutes. It will feel like an eternity so set a timer so your thoughts do not get focused on how much longer you have to sit and breathe for. The more you commit to this practice the easier and more natural it will feel.

Another easy way to get into the habit of practicing breath awareness is to choose one activity you encounter daily. For instance, you know your phone is going to ring, you are going to check your email, or social media accounts a few times throughout the day. Before you engage in this activity, pause, take a deep breath in, and slowly exhale, then move on to the activity. This brief pause helps your mind and body slow down. The subtle pause can alleviate tension and let you remain in the present moment.

Mindfulness Meditation

We discussed mindfulness practices that can help you slow down and remain present as you eat. This form of meditation can be done at any time when you need it. However, it is especially effective at interrupting thoughts of rumination or thoughts that stay stuck on past events that are causing you emotional turmoil.

When you practice mindfulness, remember to tune into all of your senses. Keep yourself in the present moment by paying particular attention to what you see and hear around you. This will help you remain calm in frustrating situations and will help reduce cravings in moments where you are mad or bored.

Movement Meditation

Yoga is one of the most commonly practiced movement meditations, though many see yoga as an exercise instead of a meditation. Movement meditation requires you to focus on your breath while performing calculated movements.

This type of meditation is effective for boosting your mood and as a relaxation technique. It is also an effective way to connect with your body.You can begin trying an easy five-minute yoga sequence to get used to inhaling and exhaling with specific body positions. You are not limited to yoga. Dancing can also transition to a type of movement meditation where you focus on how your body feels as you move, remaining in control of your breath, and keeping your thoughts in the present moment as you move.

Exercise

Exercise helps fight against emotional eating in a few key ways. First, there is plenty of research that shows exercise to be an effective way to combat stress. Sticking to a long-term exercise routine can also help reduce anxiety that can trigger emotional eating. Exercise has also been shown to help you become emotionally resilient. By exercising regularly you can handle big emotions with more clarity. Finally, exercise can help regulate your eating habits. Those who exercise are more likely to choose foods that are more nourishing over foods that provide fewer nutrients. We discuss the importance of exercise for weight loss and how to create a habit out of becoming more physical activity in the next chapter.

Journaling

Journaling is a practice that has been shown to help combat emotional stress and can be an effective way to address various eating habits you want to change. There are many journaling practices you can do that will boost your mood and bring more awareness to your daily habits from eating and exercising to sleep and negative thoughts.

One of the most recommended journaling practices that can help with emotional eating is keeping a gratitude journal. You can easily add one to three things to your journal every morning or evening that you are grateful for. It has been shown that taking a few minutes to show gratitude daily can help reduce stress and improve overall life satisfaction.

You can also keep a food journal that helps you track what you eat and why. This type of journal should not be used to restrict what or how much you eat. You do not need to count calories or ensure you are getting the right balance of macronutrients at every meal. Instead, you want to simply log what you eat and how you feel before and after you eat.

Another journal practice that can help you gain control over emotions is a thought journal. WIth this journaling practice you do a brain dump every evening to get any ruminating thoughts out of your head. You can write one thing that has been causing you stress and list possible solutions to eliminate the stress. Getting your thoughts out before you go to bed can help improve sleep as these thoughts no longer need to take up space in your mind and keep you tossing and turning throughout the night.

What To Choose

One thing to keep in mind is that you want to stick with one of the mentioned methods at a time. While it is a good idea to have a list of options, we need to retrain our brain to turn to a non-food item for comfort. Once you have been successful with handling your emotions in a different manner you can choose to utilize different activities. However, it is important to stick with just one until you feel more comfortable and confident about embracing your feelings without neglecting or numbing them.

Additionally, you do not have to choose the items mentioned here. You can try any number of activities that will help keep you in a better mood. Consider doing hobbies you enjoy, connecting with loved ones, or simply allowing yourself to rest. The best way to combat emotional eating is through self-love. When you can show yourself more loving kindness you will be more inclined to listen to what you need emotionally instead of trying to numb, ignore, or stuff down what you are feeling using food.

Chapter 7:

Getting Active

No, exercise is not a requirement. I know most of you are dreading this chapter because you dread the idea of having to workout. But, before you simply skip it and decide that working out isn't for you, pause a moment. Exercise is not punishment, it is a way for you to respect your body and optimize your health.

Exercise should be viewed as a choice you make to keep your body fit and healthy. When we begin to look at physical activity from a new perspective and change the internal dialogue around why you do not exercise, you will find that getting moving becomes enjoyable!

Despite the resistance you may have about working out, I encourage you to read through this chapter anyway. If, by the end, you still want to maintain your views about moving, then you can absolutely decide that exercise is not your thing. However, if that is what you decide today, come back to this chapter once you have begun to incorporate some healthier habits into your routines. You might find that you begin to look at exercise in a whole new way.

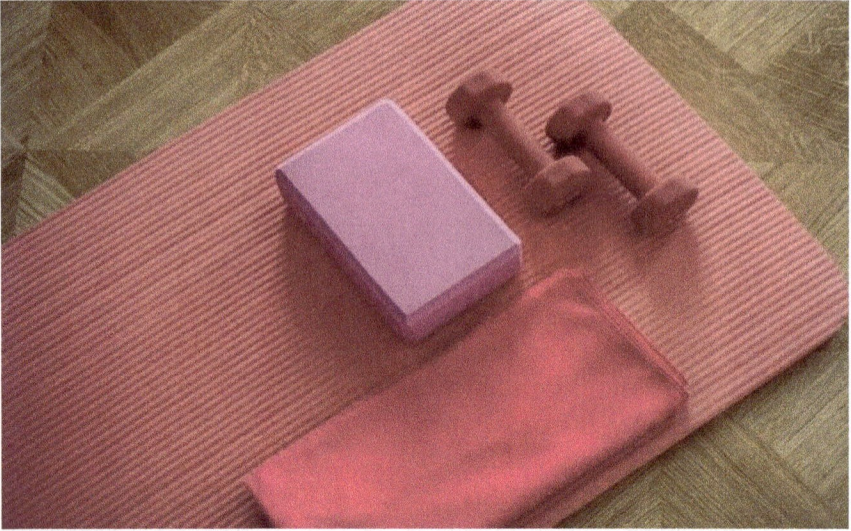

Do Not Focus on Calories Burned

The diet culture has turned exercise into an obligation and it is often perceived as a form of punishment for eating. Many people struggle to stick with exercise because they approach it only as a way to burn more calories. The many benefits regular exercise brings to your overall health is often ignored when you are trying to lose weight.

A dieting mindset looks at exercise as something you need to do so you burn more calories only. Many, once they lose the weight they want, instantly begin to slack off on their exercise and eventually stop doing it all together. They lose the motivation (weight loss) to get up and move.

The problem is that we rarely focus on what we gain from exercises. We pay more attention to what we lose and calories burned, instead of the benefits that will last a lifetime. Again, you need to focus on 'more' rather than 'less.' To make exercise a habit, start looking at it from a different perspective and attach different reasons to do it.

Why is exercise important? We already know that adequate physical activity keeps our body strong and optimally functional. However, even knowing that, millions fail to stick with or even start an exercise routine. Instead consider why it is important for you to maintain optimal health. Do you have children or grandkids you want to be able to run around and play with? Think of how being more physically fit will help you stay active in your community and volunteer for groups. What about your job? Will being more energized and strong help you keep up with a fast-paced work environment?

There are many reasons why we should exercise for our health, but when we recognize that better health allows us to do more in our lives, we are motivated to move more. We are more likely to change our habits when we recognize how our current habits hinder the relationships we have with others and our ability to fully live life the way we envision.

Ask yourself: Are you the type of person that gets moving daily or the type of person who wants to remain sedentary?

Commit to an Active Lifestyle

Dieting is likely to cause loss of muscle mass because the body will burn muscle if it is not getting adequate energy through the food you eat. This loss of muscle makes it harder to burn stored fat. Also, if you have a predominantly sedentary lifestyle, your metabolism is likely to be operating at a slower speed. These factors, plus the negative mindset you probably have around exercising make it incredibly hard to motivate yourself to move more.

When you first decide to exercise it is important that you do not put much pressure on yourself to workout for a long period of time, like 30 minutes. Nor should you force yourself to do any type of exercise you really detest. Instead of forcing yourself to get up early to workout when you are not an early riser or take a cycling class when you hate cycling, simply promise yourself to move more.

Connecting back to your compounding habits, starting a workout routine can be done the same way. So many people avoid exercising because they are out of shape and cannot complete a 30 minutes cardio session or do more than one sit-up or push-up. That is okay. If you can only walk for one minute, then commit to one minute a day. If you can only do one push-up, commit to one push-up a day.

When you decide that you are going to start being more active, add one small thing at a time. Doing one push-up a day will move you closer to your healthy lifestyle than not doing any. That one push-up can be added to, you can build upon it. Many people have started with just one: one push-up, one minute of dancing, one sit-up, one mile, a one-second plank, and so on. The one turns into two, then four, and suddenly it is a year later and you are feeling more energized, confident, and fit. One puts the wheels in motion and once you build momentum from that one thing, you begin to move and see significant changes.

After about a week or two of just doing one, you may naturally push yourself to do two. By committing to one and following through you begin to build trust in yourself which results in more willpower. When our willpower increases, so does our confidence and self-esteem. We naturally want to maintain these good feelings and are more inclined to stick with activities that induce them, such as exercising.

Learn To Love The Way You Feel

To adopt a more active lifestyle, you need to shift the way you think about exercise. Exercise is about keeping your body flexible, strong, and mobile. Physical activity should be looked at as a way to show your body respect and appreciation for all that it has done for you. You may not love the way your body looks now, but you can learn to embrace it so it continues to function the way it should for you to live a functional life.

Many of us have a poor body image, and it is difficult to take care of something if we hate or are disgusted by it. This is why you need to shift the view you have of your body and use exercise as a reward instead of a punishment. Be mindful of how you describe your workout session. Telling yourself, "I have to get up and go for a run," or "I have to go to the gym," is automatically going to cause internal resistance. Instead, try using phrases like "I get to run after work today," or "I get to start my day at the gym." This minor change from "have to" to "get to" tricks the brain into believing you are about to do something you enjoy.

Another way to motivate yourself to workout is to focus on how you feel after you move your body. We often get stuck in feeling too tired or comfortable sitting around to consider how much better we feel after we workout. Exercise increases the endorphins, which are our feel-good chemicals in the brain. We are naturally in a better mood after we get moving. Also consider how confident and unstoppable we feel after getting in a good sweat session. We need to remind ourselves how amazing we feel after we workout to push ourselves to get moving. While keeping these good feelings in the front of mind, ask yourself which is better: Sitting around feeling tired and unproductive or getting up and moving for a little while to feel more energized and ready to tackle your day?

We can also rely on how we feel to stay motivated to workout for the long-term. Instead of using the scale to track your progress, log how you feel throughout each day when you do and do not workout. Make a note of how your clothes fit. After a few weeks of sticking with an exercise routine, do you notice your clothes are fitting better or are even a little loose? These are things we want to review regularly because they have a huge impact on transforming our workouts into habits.

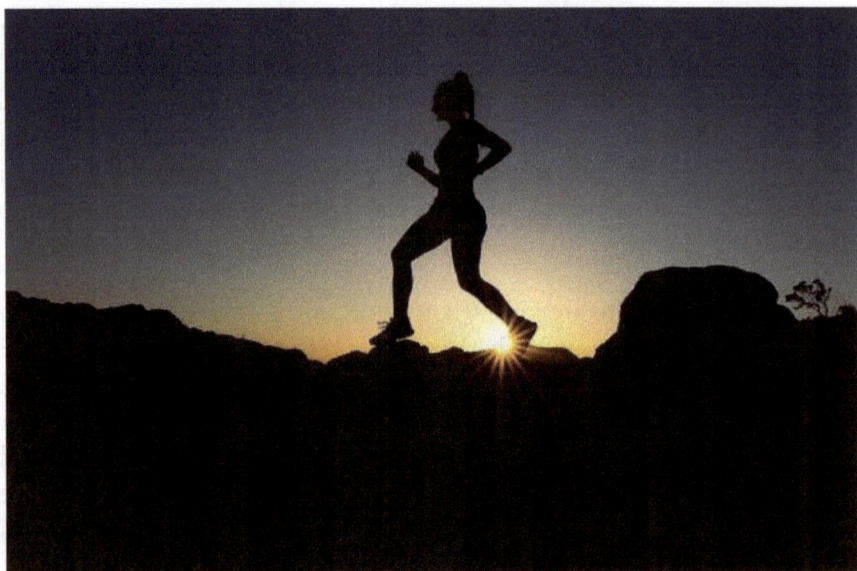

Making Physical Activity a Habit

There are some days when you are going to have to use up a lot more willpower to get moving. Other days, it will feel easy. It can be simple to stay committed for a few weeks and then life gets in the way and we begin to skip more workouts or just start sitting around more. For anything to become a habit, whether it is exercise or brushing your teeth, we need to do it consistently. To be consistent we need to make getting started as easy as possible. Below you will find a handful of helpful tips that will make moving fit seamlessly into your day so you can be consistent and reap the benefits.

Have a Ritual in Place to Make Getting Started Easier.

You can't make a habit if you do not take the steps to actually get started with the habit. Finding a way to make the initial steps easier makes creating a habit more effortless. Incorporating rituals and routines will make it easier to follow through. A ritual can be preparing your workout necessities the day before: Get your gym bag ready and set it next to the door so you can easily grab it in the morning before you leave for work. If you are exercising at home, making sure you have a clear space to work out is important

Another effective way to create a routine is to set your intentions ahead of time. Setting your intentions is as simple as filling in the following sentence:

Next week I will exercise on (DAY) at (TIME) at (PLACE).

This establishes the expectation that you will hold yourself accountable. It also takes out the guesswork of when and where you will work out. When you make the decision ahead of time you eliminate the excuse of not having time or not knowing what your exercise will consist of.

Do Not Focus on the Workout.

We are often filled with dread when we start thinking about doing a workout. We immediately begin to find excuses as to why we should skip. Instead of focusing on the workout, focus on just the quick two-minute or less task you need to accomplish to get started. Grabbing your water bottle and putting on your running shoes is a prime example. Focusing on these simple tasks can boost your motivation because you have already taken action.

Commit to Just Five Minutes.

Forcing yourself to complete a full workout when you are just not feeling it will not result in being eager to do it again. Your brain will register your dislike and frustration as something it needs to avoid in the future, which only makes it harder. There are going to be days where you just need to give yourself some grace, tell yourself you will do just five minutes. If after five minutes you are still not into the workout, allow yourself to stop. What most people find is that once they have gone through the first five minutes they stick it out for another five minutes, or fifteen minutes, or more.

Do Not Focus on the Results.

It is easy to get discouraged when you are trying to do something to improve your health or lose weight and do not see immediate results. Most people try to start an exercise habit by creating a goal that has a definitive end. "I want to lose 10 pounds." What often occurs is when they fail to lose the desired amount of weight they look at their efforts as wasted time and energy.

It is the process we want to focus on. Remember, habits help us form new identities. Are you the type of person that values their physical health and therefore doesn't miss a workout? This is what you want to focus on.

Once you have established a consistent routine then you can focus on progress, or the result you seek. By establishing the routine first, the results will naturally follow, and then you shift your focus to improving. Your workout becomes a way of becoming stronger, building endurance, and pushing yourself. Unless the habits have become a part of your routine you have nothing to build on and, no matter what strategy you try to use, the results will not last.

Physical Activity Suggestions

There are many ways you can move more throughout the day without having to call it an exercise or workout session. The goal is to make physical activity a part of your lifestyle and this doesn't have to mean running five times a week or lifting weights twice a week. You already know you can run, bike, and swim to get in a good workout but consider the following activities that will get you moving more, too.

- gardening

- mowing the lawn

- raking leaves

- shoveling snow

- parking further from entrances

- using a standing desk

- disembarking one stop early on public transportation and walking

- playing community sports

- coaching your child's activities

- in the office, walking to speak to your coworkers instead of emailing or texting

- taking a movement break every 50 minutes

- doing activities you enjoyed as a child playing with your your kids outdoors

- walking your dog

- walking as you talk on the phone

- parking down the block when picking your kids up from school and walking to greet them

Physical activity does not have to be as structured as many believe it should be. You can probably find plenty of ways to move a little more during your day. Remember that moving more should be something you enjoy. Even a little extra movement can help you feel better and move more easily and, if you stick with it, you will benefit from the compound effect.

Chapter 8:

Goal Setting for Weight Loss

Traditional goal setting will not help you create better habits to lose weight. Many people do recommend setting one specific goal, which can be highly effective, but for creating a habit to build upon you need to do more than just set a goal. Remember, you are making life-long changes. Most goals are established to be achieved and then forgotten. You are simply encouraged to set another goal. You do not want to get to an end result. Instead, you want to establish goals that allow continuous progress.

If you are like most, you have probably set a number of goals that focus on weight loss. Have you set New Year's resolutions and after a few weeks quickly forgot them? The problem is, that most people set the wrong goals. They focus on the outcome and not the process. If we set goals in this manner we are not likely to stay motivated. Creating habits is not just about changing your behaviors but it is about becoming the person you know you are capable of being. Who you become in the process is what will serve as your motivation. This is important to keep in mind as you begin to establish goals for your weight loss journey.

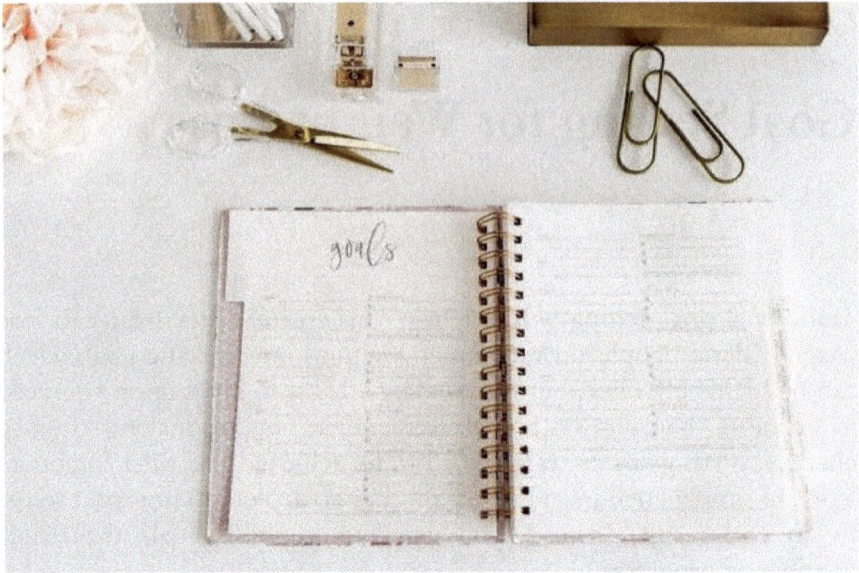

Effective Goals

Solid goals will provide you with the strategy to get you to the healthy lifestyle you desire. Remember, having the right mindset is essential for making progress. After that, losing weight and taking control of your health becomes an enjoyable process because you should not be focusing on dropping pounds. Goals for weight loss should revolve around adopting the right habits and behaviors. Otherwise, you will return to your old ways of eating.

Before setting any goal, it is vital that you understand what you want by achieving the goals. Goals that are set to accomplish short-term victories will not result in long-lasting changes. While short-term goals can help motivate you at first, they will not keep you dedicated to forming the habits that will improve your life for the long run. For example, many people set goals based on upcoming events. You want to look good in your wedding dress or swimsuit. There is a reunion coming up or a work party at which you are receiving an award and you want to look your best. What happens after the event has passed? You abandon the daily actions that got you down to a smaller size and let you glow on your big night.

It is great to use short-term goals to get you started but you need to dig deeper to stay committed beyond that. Consider what else you will gain from creating your new habits. Ultimately, do you want to feel more confident? If you have children wouldn't you rather be able to keep up with them instead of sitting on the sidelines? Consider all the things improving your health will provide you. The intrinsic motivation that comes from within will keep you aligned and on track with making the necessary changes you desire.

Many people recommend creating SMART goals when trying to lose weight. If your goal is only to lose weight this can be effective. SMART goals check off the following items:

- Specific

- Measurable

- Actionable

- Realistic/relatable

- Time-bound

Unfortunately, many people who have struggled with their weight find that setting goals in this manner do not provide them with the results they initially set out to achieve. This is often due to setting goals based on the dieting mindset: "I need to lose X amount of weight by this day." If you do not lose that much weight, you feel defeated. Additionally, the most common way people tend to measure these goals is by tracking their weight, how much they exercise, or how many inches they lose. These measurable items all feed into the dieting mindset.

Instead, shift your focus from the external to the internal and find long-term solutions rather than temporary fixes. We want to ensure that we are implementing the habits that will lead to natural weight loss and have you feeling more energized and healthy. When you set goals for weight loss, your focus should be on the daily actions we want to perform. Goals should check off the following components.

Simple

You want to build on top of your goals. Remember we are forming new habits, not temporary changes. Avoid setting goals that can't be expanded, added too, or maintained once you hit them.

Actionable

You need to identify the first steps that you need to take. Break down your bigger goals into steps that are easy to achieve. Your efforts will compound so do not think that your goal is too small or that you need to be doing more. So set goals you know you will achieve and do not set any goals that you have been told you should do.

Realistic

If you are not confident in your ability to follow through on the steps or reach your goal, you will not stay committed. Many people are overly enthusiastic about setting their healthy lifestyle goals, which is not always a bad thing, however most people mistakenly think they need to make monumental changes in a short amount of time.

Consider Obstacles

Consider how you may get off track and formulate a plan to address obstacles before you have to face them. For example, you may tell yourself that you are going to eat from the salad bar at work for lunch every day instead of ordering out or grabbing something from the local fast food chain. But, everyday at lunch you get to the salad bar and the lettuce is wilted and you have few options for toppings. You are determined to stick with your initial goal of eating at that salad bar, but conditions outside of your control are making that very difficult.

You need another option to help you achieve your goals. You may need to make adjustments as you go, as we can't always foresee obstacles until they are right in front of us. Remember to be flexible.Just because something stands in your way or gets you off course one day does not mean you have to give up entirely. A healthy lifestyle will be a process that you will continuously adjust as you go through different phases of your life.

Action Plan Examples

Use the following as a guide to help you establish your own goals. Each example provides a goal. This is the end goal you want to eventually reach. There is no set time frame for accomplishing it. The only thing you need to do is commit to making consistent action. Under each goal you will find an action plan. This plan provides several suggestions for how to implement the necessary changes and options for building on top of certain steps. You do not have to follow this action plan as it is outlined. Instead, you can choose one action item to start with and complete them in any order you desire.

Goal: Drink 100 ounces of water a day.

Action Plan:

- Track your water intake and track when you drink other beverages to see where you might add in water down the road. This will give you an honest look at where you are starting.

- Drink water first thing in the morning,

- Have water with your lunch before you reach for the soda.

- Carry water around with you and sip on it throughout the day.

- Start your meals with a glass of water.

- When you feel the urge to snack on something, drink water first. If you are still hungry 10 minutes later then eat.

Your goal may be to drink more water, eat a well-balanced breakfast, get proper sleep, or move your body more. All these goals can have a limitation and will naturally wean out some of the unwanted behaviors.

Goal: Eat breakfast daily.

Action Plan:

- If you never eat breakfast, simply begin by having a piece of fruit or yogurt to start your day.

- Have three to five go to breakfast recipes that you can make ahead and grab and go in the morning.

- Eating a balanced breakfast just one day a week. This meal consists of lean protein, a little fat, and whole -grains. For example, scramble eggs with onions and mushrooms wrapped in a whole-wheat tortilla.

- Plan your breakfasts for three days a week.

Goal: Sleep eight hours every night.

Action Plan:

- Stop drinking caffeine by 2:00 p.m.

- Create a sleep environment.

- Stop using electronics at least one hour before bed.

- Do a relaxing yoga sequence an hour before bed.

- Create an evening routine that encourages sleep.

- Create a morning routine where you are excited to jump out of bed to start.

- Wake up at the same time everyday, even on the weekends.

- Journal before bed to get out any stressful thoughts.

- Create a to-do list for the next day in the evening.

- Ensure there is proper air circulation in your bedroom.

- Lower the temperature slightly.

Goal: Work out five days a week for 30 minutes.

Action Plan:

- Track what you do throughout the day. This will provide you with a clear schedule that will help you add in more physical activity.

- Walk for five minutes every morning or evening.

- Stretch first thing in the morning.

- Add exercise where you can. Take the stairs more, do a few squats as you fold laundry, turn on some music and dance as you wash the dishes.

- Try a new type of exercise once a month.

- Plan what you will do if the weather does not allow you to get outside or if another change in your schedule requires you to rework your physical activity times.

- Commit to just five minutes of physical activity a day. Then add five minutes at a time.

- Incorporate different types of physical activity. Add a strength training day. If you tend to walk or jog, try swimming or biking one day. Mixing it up will keep things interesting.

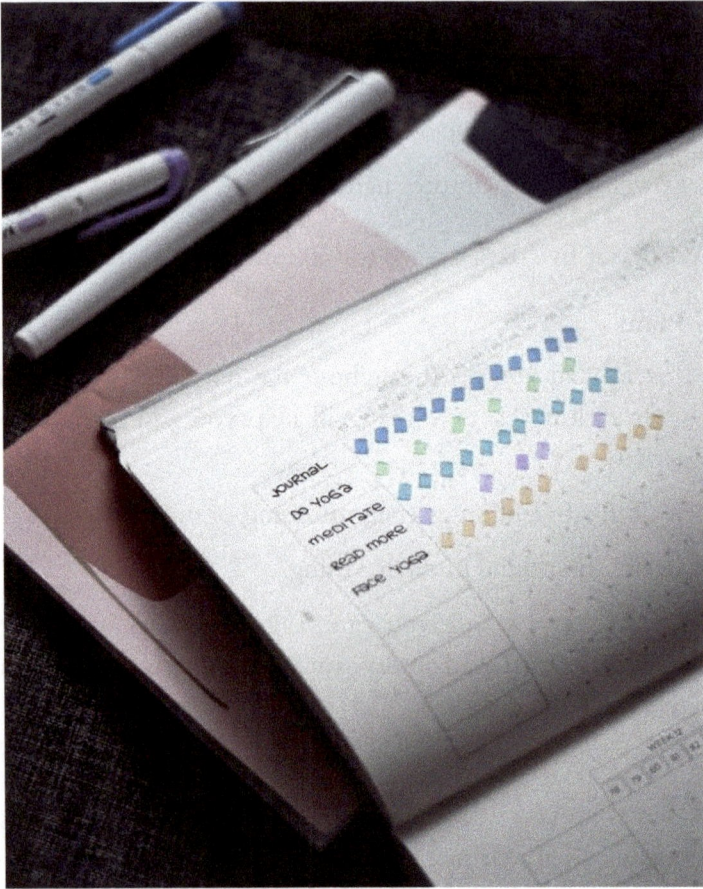

Review and Scale

Do not set yourself up for failure by adding another action or building on a current one before you are ready. This is what holds many people back. They want to rush to the end so they overcommit themselves. Research has shown that a steady approach to weight loss is likely to lead to keeping the weight off.

Reviewing progress is essential. You need to know that your efforts are paying off but, more importantly, you need to know when you are getting off track. There are many reasons why you may not be sticking to your new habit routine; often it is because you are trying to make something stick that is not the right fit. Remember, there is no one-size-fits-all approach to creating a healthy lifestyle or losing weight. Everyone is different and your lifestyle may not allow you to hit the gym five days a week or cook dinner every night. You need to learn how to be flexible with your approach to get the results you want and can sustain.

Only by tracking and reviewing progress will you uncover where and why your new habits are not working. For example, you may have set a goal to run three days a week after work. Upon reviewing, you realize you have only been running one day a week because the other days you get home too late and heading outside to run is not an option. Without reviewing you may have thought that you were making great progress, and get frustrated later on when your results do not add up to what you feel they should be. It is easy for us to tell ourselves repeatedly, "At least I got in one day," and be satisfied. You may tell yourself week after week, "I will stick to all three days next week." But months go by and you do not realize how long you have been putting off running all three days.

You may continue to make progress by running one or two days a week, however if you are tracking and reviewing you will identify this issue. You can decide to run in the morning or in the afternoon. You might swap two of your running days for an indoor cardio session at home instead. This is why reviewing is essential for progress. If you simply continue to stick with a routine that is not working for you, you will continue to be disappointed with your results.

On the other end of the spectrum, what happens when you have been sticking with your action steps but have stopped seeing progress? When we have been putting in our best efforts and at first saw great results, not seeing these results weeks later can stifle motivation. In this instance, your actions need to be reviewed so you alter or add to them and break through your plateau.

One thing that is often ignored is what happens when you reach your goals. Maybe you have reached your set goal and need to make room in your schedule to set other goals. Sometimes sticking with your current routine may not allow for additional goals to be put into action. When this occurs, many people tend to stop doing what gave them the results, which often leads to returning to old ways and being disappointed when the weight comes back or our health takes a dip into the negative. It is important to know how and when to scale back on some habits. You do not want to completely stop what has gotten you to where you are, but there is also a time where there is no need to continue building or adding on. For example, you set a goal to eat plant-based five days a week. You have reached your goal, you feel great, but you want to keep those other two days free for more flexibility with what you eat. You also have realized that, while you like eating a plant-based diet, you want to incorporate some other foods during the week like eggs for breakfast or fish one day a week. In this case you would scale back on your habit. You still want to continue eating plant-based but also want to have more variety in the foods you eat for health benefits.

Scaling back is not about adding in habits that do not benefit your health. It is reevaluating your goals and knowing that they are allowed to change so you continue to make progress. It is also understanding that once you reach your peak, you do not need to keep adding more. Once you hit your goal of working out for 30 minutes five days a week, you do not have to add on another day or more time. If you are satisfied with that goal and it is something you can comfortably maintain you do not have to keep building on it.

Question for reviewing goal:

- What are my wins or what is working?
- What obstacles have I encountered?
- What have I enjoyed?
- What hasn't been working?
- Have I been honest with my tracking?
- What upcoming events might get in the way of sticking to my current routine?

- Is what I am doing too easy or too hard?

- How do I need to make adjustments to further my progress?

- What do I need to readjust so I can better commit to my action plan?

Remember, reviewing your goals and progress is not about feeling guilty if you have not stuck with your original plan. Always give yourself grace. Adopting a healthy lifestyle is a process. Focus on what has been working and change what hasn't. Make it a habit to review your progress weekly. This will let you see where you are slacking off and quickly make adjustments for the upcoming week. Schedule time to do a more thorough review of your goals once a month. This will allow you to make adjustments to your action plan to ensure you continue with your progress.

Chapter 9:

Accountability

We are more likely to follow through and achieve our goals when we hold ourselves accountable to others. If we learn to hold ourselves accountable to ourselves, we will rise above the expectation we have for ourselves. Unfortunately, it is easier f to abandon promises we make to ourselves than to disappoint others. Keeping yourself on track is essential because if we want to create a habit we need to be consistent with our efforts.

Finding an accountability partner is one of the most common ways to help stay on track. But they can also keep us off track. You may not have the right people around you that you are willing to turn to for support. There are other options for keeping yourself accountable that you may want to consider.

How to Keep Yourself Accountable

Keeping yourself accountable will ensure that you stay committed to making the changes you desire. Following through on the things you said you would require proper management of your time, energy, and task. It is not easy for many people to hold themselves accountable when it comes to losing weight or adopting healthier habits. Too many temptations distract us from our goals and we encounter too many days where we forget why we said we want to lose weight to begin with.

In the beginning of your weight loss journey, having someone to keep you on track can be essential for your success. Once you have become comfortable with your new habits you will need to rely less and less on others to hold you accountable. Also, once you have gone through the process of starting small and slowly making changes it will become easier to hold yourself accountable because you have more trust in yourself to follow through on your commitments to yourself.

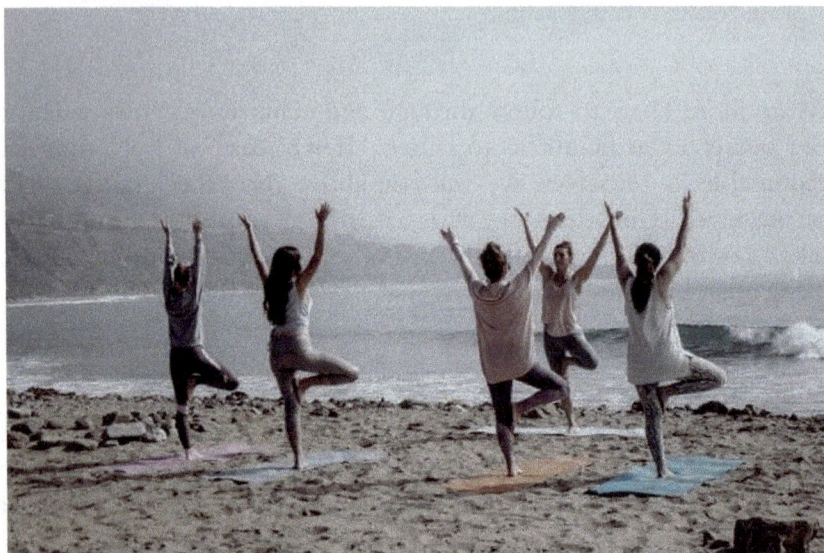

Accountability Partner

An accountability partner is highly recommended if you struggle with self-motivation. However, you can't pick just anyone to hold you accountable. There are times when having an accountability partner can hinder your progress and they may even unintentionally cause you to give up on your goals.

Before choosing an accountability partner is it important that your own goals are clear to you. You can't ask someone to help you stay on track if you are not clear about what you need help staying accountable to. Whether it is your eating habits or exercise habits, know specifically what you need to be doing so your partner will know what to ask to ensure you are sticking to your goals.

After you have decided what you need from your accountability partner, you need to choose one carefully. Would it be in your best interest to ask someone to hold you accountable if they are unreliable? An accountability person needs to be someone on whom you know you can depend. Some things to consider when looking for an accountability partner:

- Do they have the time? Anyone can agree to be an accountability partner, especially if they are not aware of the time commitment they are agreeing to. We all have busy lives and your partner should have the time and be just as invested in seeing you accomplish your goals as you are. Discuss both your schedule to decide when you both can meet regularly to check in. If you expect them to join you in a workout or two during the week, these times also have to be arranged. It will not do you any good if your partner needs to constantly cancel or reschedule meetings.

- Are they more disciplined than you? It is in your best interest to find a partner who is more disciplined than you. One that has also gone through and achieved what you are trying to do is also beneficial, though not a requirement. Having a partner that you know always follows through on their own commitments is one that you can expect to push you to follow through on your commitments. Those who are more disciplined tend to put up with fewer excuses and will be more honest when you both know you are only putting in half the effort.

- Who is someone you can't stand the thought of disappointing? You may easily break promises you make to yourself. How many times have you told yourself you were going to start taking your health more seriously, but something always came up that didn't allow for you to follow through? It is much harder for us to break the promises we make to others. If you know someone you would hate to let down or have to say, "I haven't gotten to it yet" when you promised you would, this is an ideal candidate to have as an accountability partner.

- Do not limit yourself to just one person. You might be hesitant to choose more than one accountability partner but not every partnership is going to make it. It is better to reach out to a few people so you have more people to answer to. Imagine having to tell multiple people you didn't workout or you haven't been eating according to your plan.

- You also have to keep them accountable. A partnership is two ways. You need to consider that just as you are expecting your partner to keep you on track you need to know how you can help keep them on track. Even if they are further along than you in adopting a healthier lifestyle, it is important that you give in this arrangement as well. If your partner is insistent on not needing to be held accountable then ensure that you are counting on them to hold you accountable. It can be easy for others not to put much weight on keeping another person on track, and this can lead to missing check-in or update meetings.

You want to ensure the person you embark on this journey with is someone you trust to be straightforward with you to keep you on track. It needs to be someone who is willing to put in the effort to ensure you are getting up to do your workout but do not expect them to hold your hand the entire way.

If you can't find someone among your friends, consider online communities. Having social support has been shown to help individuals stick to their goals. Online support groups can provide the accountability you are seeking from someone in-person. Online groups and communities allow you to share your progress and struggles, so you never feel alone in your journey.

Tracking

You can't change what you do not track. Tracking is a great way to keep yourself accountable. Having your habits scheduled into your day, just as you schedule doctor appointments, will better ensure you commit to them. Tracking what you do lets you see the progress you are making, or lets you honestly uncover when you are skipping a few too many days.

It can be easy to let one rest day turn into two, then a week, and then a month. Tracking gives you an easy-to-see glimpse at the work you are or are not doing. There are various apps that help let you log your workouts, meals, sleep, meditation, and any other habit you are trying to make stick. You can just as easily keep a journal to record your efforts.

Aside from tracking what you are doing it is also encouraged that you take pictures or measurements as you get started on your journey. 'Goodbye' or 'before' photos provide a visual of where you are starting. These images are just pictures taken from the front and side on the first day you begin your new habit. Then every three to four weeks you take another set.

These images should provide extra motivation to keep going. It can be hard to see the changes your body is going through when you look at yourself everyday in the mirror. When you take images and compare them you see the evidence of your hard work.

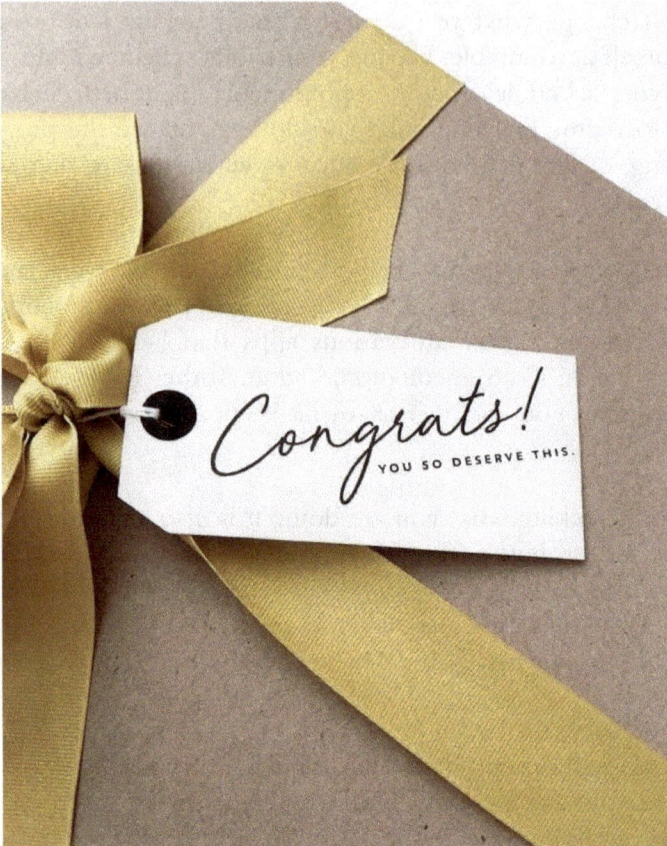

It is vital that you celebrate your progress or your self-motivation will diminish. Having the right reward in place can increase your chances of sticking to your healthy routines. Many fall into the trap of allowing themselves a 'cheat' day or a food reward for doing such a great job sticking to their new habits. However, this can be counterproductive, as one reward turns into two and then many more which begins to hinder your progress.

Instead of using food as a reward for your success, whether it be weight loss or any other area in your life, find other incentives to keep you motivated. Think of something special you can do for yourself, such as a trip to the spa or a new haircut. Or consider the things you enjoy to buy occasionally for yourself like candles, bath bombs, or books. You can set up little rewards for each week you stay committed.

Some other ideas for treating yourself include:

- Get a facial

- Get a manicure

- Buy a new pair of running shoes

- A trip to the movies

- Buy new makeup

- Buy yourself concert tickets

- Buy a new outfit

- Buy yourself flowers

- Purchase new workout equipment

- Buy something to use in the kitchen to help you plan or prep your meals.

You can also start a reward jar. If there is a big purchase you want to make like buying a smartwatch or taking a mini vacation this is a good idea to help you save while you stay committed to your goals. Set the jar out next to a picture of what you want or a sign that reminds you what it is for. Every time you stick to your new habit add a little change to the jar.

What if Nothing Is Working?

Sometimes you can try everything in your power to stick to a healthier lifestyle but still find yourself performing old unwanted habits. What you need to understand is that a healthy lifestyle is not a solo journey. Everyone needs support as they make their transition to better habits and they need encouragement to stay with them. Even so, you may have all the support you need and still find yourself hiding disordered eating habits or feeling a lack of motivation constantly to get up and get moving.

You may want to consider reaching out for additional professional help. Before you start thinking it is weak or pathetic to have to seek out help, understand that you are not alone in your struggles. Over 28 million people in the US alone report to have an eating disorder that hinders them from living a healthier lifestyle (Eating Disorder Statistics, n.d.). Keep in mind, this is only the number of people that report having serious issues with their eating habits and weight, millions of other people keep their conditions hidden.

It is not weak to ask for help. It is much better to get help to create the changes you desire than to continue to suffer and struggle in silence. Also, know that help can come in many forms. Some people find reaching out to the doctor to find someone to help them create healthy eating plans is better for them. Others find that they need more support or accountability with the exercises. Do not think that asking for help means you have failed, instead look at is a way to ensure you succeed. Some professionals you might want to consider are discussed below.

Nutritionist or Dietitian

Both a nutritionist and dietitian can help you adopt a new approach to eating. Dietitians are certified to treat specific conditions from diabetes to eating disorders. Nutritionists do not have to be certified but, if you choose to work with one, we recommend you choose one who does hold some kind of training and certification. Nutritionists often have more specific areas of focus than dietitians, such as sport nutrition or autoimmune condition nutrition.

Dietitians and nutritionists can help you gain a better understanding of what makes up a healthy diet, how to better prepare and plan meals to the appropriate portions, and how to schedule your meals so you are providing your body with optimal nutrition throughout the day.

Medical Nutrition Therapy

During medical nutrition therapy, you work with a registered dietitian or a registered dietitian nutritionist. This therapy discusses your current eating habits and diet. You work with the dietitian to set realistic goals, many of which we have covered throughout this book, like drinking more water and increasing physical activity. They help you create a plan that you can stick with and that works for your lifestyle. If you find that you are lacking the motivation or still feel overwhelmed trying to adopt new habits on your own, this can be a highly effective way to help you change for the better.

Personal Trainer

A personal trainer can be useful if you need extra motivation to get more active. Personal trainers are also beneficial because they guide you through different types of workouts and ensure that you have the correct form to minimize injury. When you find the right trainer, they will help you find the best type of exercise to get you the results you desire. Professional trainers have a deeper understanding of what muscle groups to activate to burn fat. They can help you create a workout plan best suited for your current activity levels and teach you the best way to increase your physical activity for long-term results. This can be especially beneficial for those that may suffer from injuries. A personal trainer will teach you how to modify your workouts so they are still effective at helping you lose weight and maintain an active lifestyle.

Behavioral Therapy

Many find that behavioral therapy helps them address the root cause of their unhealthy habits. With this therapy approach, you uncover and address the thought patterns and behaviors that lead to emotional, binge, and other eating disorders. When you work with a trained therapist they can help you find flaws in the way you think about yourself and your ability to live a healthier lifestyle. They work with you to establish goals that are based around your behaviors as opposed to what or how much you eat.

A behavioral therapist can work with you to address various elements of your lifestyle. They guide you to identify what you think is keeping you from a healthy weight and work with you to improve your body image and combat limiting beliefs. This is an effective strategy to overcome disordered eating habits that are deeply ingrained into your daily living. It takes time to rewire some of the thoughts and opinions you have around food and what is considered 'healthy' eating. Your therapist will help you remain focused on your desired goals. Once you have reached your main health goals, they will help you establish a plan to maintain your results.

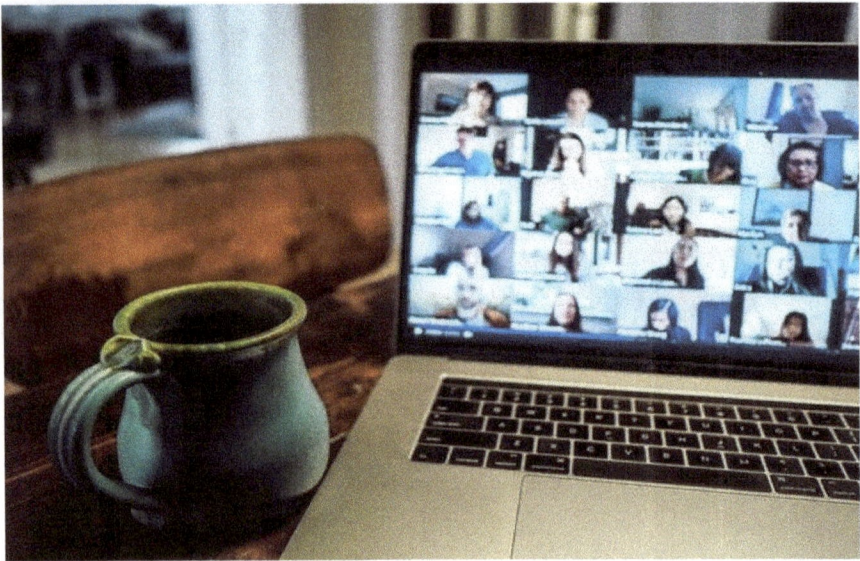

Conclusion

When you struggle with being overweight it can leave you desperate for a solution that works, and works quickly with little effort. It is why many of us follow one diet after another in hopes that the next one will finally be the one that keeps the weight off. Unfortunately, the damage you are causing by yo-yo dieting and following fad diets is only going to cause you to gain more weight over the long-term.

You picked up this book because you were looking for a more effective approach to help you lose weight and finally keep it off. What you have gained is a new perspective on how to approach weight loss. You have thought for so long that if you just eat a certain way and work out a little you will achieve the results you desire. While you may have reached goals temporarily, you were not able to sustain them.

This book has walked you through the process of creating habits that will result in a healthier lifestyle. You have learned why you need to reframe how you think about food, your body, and exercise. Action steps are provided that show you how to begin incorporating the core healthy eating habits that will lead to weight loss. You now know how to create effective goals that you can finally follow through on. Once you accomplish these goals, you understand how to continue to build on them for long-term results.

If there is anything you should take away from this book, it is that you begin to trust your body. That you learn to honor the hunger and fullness cues it sends you. That you see yourself as a beautiful person worthy of respect and love. I hope that you use the advice provided throughout this book to show your body love and respect by choosing to nourish it and keep it active.

The goal of this book was to provide you with a more effective way to manage your way. A way that helps you align with what your body is naturally designed to do. It is my hope that you realize you do not have to over complicate your efforts. You do not have to go all in; things do not have to be all or nothing. You can enjoy your food, you can love the way your body moves, and you can achieve a weight that you feel confident and happy with.

I hope that, starting today, you stop focusing on the pounds you lose and instead begin to enjoy the journey you are on. A journey to a healthier and happier you! Now that you have the tools to get started on that, it is up to you to take that first small step. Start today, and you will be amazed by how much you change by deciding to commit to that one small change. Remember, weight loss is not a sprint. There is no one-size-fits all approach to losing weight. Choose the most effective first step that is right for you and remain patient. In time, the small efforts will add up.

I thank you for allowing me to be your guide on this new lifestyle. If you have found value in what you learned, share it with your friends and family. Leave a review and share with others how this information has allowed you to transform your life. I wish you luck as you continue on your path.

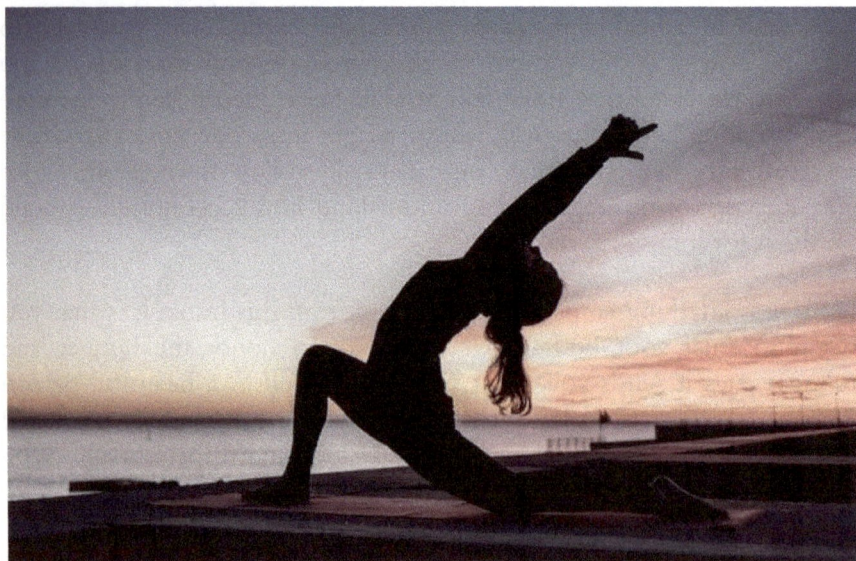

References

Alexander, H. (n.d.). *Does your body have a set point weight and can you change it?* MD Anderson Cancer Center. https://www.mdanderson.org/publications/focused-on-health/what-is-your-body-s-set-point-weight-and-can-you-change-it-.h15-1593780.html

Boschmann, M., Steiniger, J., Hille, U., Tank, J., Adams, F., Sharma, A. M., Klaus, S., Luft, F. C., & Jordan, J. (2003). Water-induced thermogenesis. The Journal of Clinical Endocrinology and Metabolism, 88(12), 6015–6019. https://doi.org/10.1210/jc.2003-030780

Clear, J. (n.d.-a). *3 simple ways to make exercise a habit.* James Clear. https://jamesclear.com/exercise-habit

Clear, J. (n.d.-b). *Habit stacking: How to build new habits by taking advantage of old ones.* James Clear. https://jamesclear.com/habit-stacking

Cognitive behavioral therapy for weight loss (CBT). (n.d.). MyVMC. https://www.myvmc.com/banners-weight-loss-centre/cognitive-behavioural-therapy-for-weight-loss-cbt/

Cooper, J. (2021, June 13). *Do I need a nutritionist or dietitian?* WebMD. https://www.webmd.com/diabetes/nutritionist-dietitian-choose

Discovery Contributor. (n.d.). *Did my mom cause my eating disorder? Six ways parents unintentionally teach disordered eating to their children.* Center for Discovery. https://centerfordiscovery.com/blog/mom-cause-eating-disorder-six-ways-parents-unintentionally-teach-disordered-eating-children/

Eating disorder statistics. (n.d.). ANAD. https://anad.org/eating-disorders-statistics/

Elliott, B. (2020, September 9). *17 Creative ways to eat more vegetables.* Healthline. https://www.healthline.com/nutrition/17-ways-to-eat-more-veggies#TOC_TITLE_HDR_19

Ellis, E. (2020, December 1). *How to add whole grains to your diet.* Eat Right Academy of Nutrition and Dietetics. https://www.eatright.org/food/nutrition/dietary-guidelines-and-myplate/how-to-add-whole-grains-to-your-diet

Floyd, S. (2016, March 2). *5 Tips for choosing the best accountability partner.* Black Enterprise. https://www.blackenterprise.com/5-tips-for-choosing-the-best-accountability-partner/

Frey, M. (2021, January 27). *Protein for weight loss: High protein foods lists, diet tips, and recipes.* Very well Fit. https://www.verywellfit.com/how-to-lose-weight-with-lean-protein-3495933

Gold, G. (2016, April 4). *7 common bad eating habits—and how To finally kick them.* SELF. https://www.self.com/story/7-common-bad-eating-habits-and-how-to-finally-kick-them

Halland, B. (n.d.). *6 Meditations to curb emotional eating.* Thrive. https://thriveglobal.com/stories/6-meditations-to-curb-emotional-eating/

Laurence, E. (2021, September 16). *When you eat directly affects your circadian rhythm and sleep quality-Here's how.* Well+Good. https://www.wellandgood.com/mealtime-sleep/

Nicholas, H. (2017, February 9). *Whole grains increase metabolism, may help promote weight loss.* Medical News Today. https://www.medicalnewstoday.com/articles/315744#Eating-fiber-in-whole-grains-increased-calories-lost-per-day

Pietrangelo, A. (2022, March 18). *Saturated vs. unsaturated fat*. Healthline. https://www.healthline.com/health/food-nutrition/saturated-and-unsaturated-fat#saturated-fat

Reiland, L. (2021, July 12). *Tips for drinking more water*. Mayo Clinic Health System. https://www.mayoclinichealthsystem.org/hometown-health/speaking-of-health/tips-for-drinking-more-water

Rumsey, A. (n.d.). *The hunger-fullness scale*. Alissa Rumsey. https://alissarumsey.com/hunger-fullness-scale/

Spritzler, F. (2021, May 21). *14 Easy ways to increase your protein intake*. Healthline. https://www.healthline.com/nutrition/14-ways-to-increase-protein-intake#TOC_TITLE_HDR_10

Study finds difference between mindless and distracted eating. (2020, April 30). University of Pittsburgh: Pittwire. https://www.pitt.edu/pittwire/features-articles/study-finds-difference-between-mindless-and-distracted-eating#:~:text=%E2%80%9CMindless%20eating%20occurs%20when%20you

The Open University. (n.d.). *Nutrition Module: 2. Nutrients and their sources*. Open.edu. https://www.open.edu/openlearncreate/mod/oucontent/view.php?id=315&printable=1

Vitamin and minerals: Are you getting what you need? (n.d.). HelpGuide. https://www.helpguide.org/harvard/vitamins-and-minerals.htm

Weight loss—A healthy approach. (n.d.). Better Health Channel. https://www.betterhealth.vic.gov.au/health/healthyliving/weight-loss-a-healthy-approach

Weight loss: How to reset your brain for success. (2021, December 30). Health Essentials from Cleveland Clinic. https://health.clevelandclinic.org/this-is-your-brain-on-a-diet/

Why diets don't work: How to avoid the dieting cycle & eat for your health. (2019, February 28). Mercy Cedar Rapids. https://www.mercycare.org/services/food-nutrition/why-diets-dont-work/

Photography References

Garrett, K. (2018, December 19). Group yoga session on the beach {digital image}. Retrieved from Unsplash https://unsplash.com/photos/GaprWyIw66o

Jimmy Dean. (2020, November, 30). Huge selection of foods {digital image}. Retrieved from Unsplash https://unsplash.com/photos/Yn0l7uwBrpw

Kloppenburg, E. (2020, June 4). Pink exercise mat with weights {digital image}. Retrieved from Unsplash https://unsplash.com/photos/erUC4fTtCuo

Lark, B. (2017, May 10). Fruit bowl and oversized tea cup {digital image}. Retrieved from Unsplash https://unsplash.com/photos/nTZOILVZuOg

Morales, J. (2020, December 19). White coffee cup {digital image}. Retrieved from Unsplash https://unsplash.com/photos/foeTT7H7SuA

Montgomery, C. (2020, April 29). Zoom call with coffee {digital image}. Retrieved from Unsplash https://unsplash.com/photos/smgTvepind4

Nascimento, B. (2016, October 14). Walking up stairs {digital image}. Retrieved from Unsplash https://unsplash.com/photos/PHIgYUGQPvU

Nik (2021, April 3). Sad, happy, angry faces drawn on eggs {digital image}. Retrieved from Unsplash https://unsplash.com/photos/iMwgWUbXxms

No Revisions (2020, November 22). Group of people sharing a large pizza and cans of pop. {digital image}. Retrieved from Unsplash https://unsplash.com/photos/jCvbQdgHxFo

Polekhina, D. (2021, January, 19). *Fork with measuring tape* {digital image}. Retrieved from Unsplash https://unsplash.com/photos/OpB7gkQY9oc.

Prophesee Journals. (2019, September 23). Habit tracker {digital image}. Retrieved from Unsplash https://unsplash.com/photos/WI30grRfBnE

Rice, J. (2017, September, 22). Women meditation in sunlight {digital image}. Retrieved from Unsplash https://unsplash.com/photos/NTyBbu66_SI

Thought Catalog. (2018, July 18). *The empty hungry plate* {digital image}.Retrieved from Unsplash https://unsplash.com/photos/fnztlIb52gU.

Tofoya, C. (2020, May 20). Congrats gifts {digital image}. Retrieved from Unsplash https://unsplash.com/photos/_Q0dP8xiUGA

Trovato, G. (2021, February 15). Glass of ice water {digital image}. Retrieved from Unsplash https://unsplash.com/photos/a23kzOSpv2Y

Vega, K. (2018, December 9). Woman doing yoga {digital image}. Retrieved from Unsplash https://unsplash.com/photos/F2qh3yjz6Jk

Venti Views. (2020, July 16). Women running on a trail. {digital image}. Retrieved from Unsplash https://unsplash.com/photos/I1EWTM5mFEM

Vittoriosi, E. (2018, June 11). Bowl of chips {digital image}. Retrieved from Unspalshhttps://unsplash.com/photos/ONQ86GlHs3c

Williams, A. (2019, July 4). Goal planner {digital image}. Retrieved from Unsplash https://unsplash.com/photos/YwBX02K60A4

Yunmai, I. (2018 April, 4). Standing on a scale {digital image}. Retrieved from Unsplash https://unsplash.com/photos/5jctAMjz21A

www.ingramcontent.com/pod-product-compliance
Lightning Source LLC
Chambersburg PA
CBHW072106040426
42334CB00042B/2492